100 WALKS IN

WEST SUSSEX

NATALIE LEAL

 THE CROWOOD PRESS

First published in 2023 by
The Crowood Press Ltd
Ramsbury, Marlborough
Wiltshire SN8 2HR

enquiries@crowood.com
www.crowood.com

British Library Cataloguing-in-Publication Data
A catalogue record for this book is available from the British Library.

ISBN 978 0 7198 4195 8

Mapping in this book is sourced from the following products: OS Explorer OL08, OL10,
OL11, OL33, OL34; OS Landranger 187, 197, 198
© Crown copyright 2016 Ordnance Survey. Licence number 100038003

Every effort has been made to ensure the accuracy of this book. However, changes can
occur during the lifetime of an edition. The Publishers cannot be held responsible for any
errors or omissions or for the consequences of any reliance on the information given in
this book, but should be very grateful if walkers could let us know of any inaccuracies by
writing to us at the address above or via the website.

As with any outdoor activity, accidents and injury can occur. We strongly advise
readers to check the local weather forecast before setting out and to take an OS map.
The Publishers accept no responsibility for any injuries which may occur in relation to
following the walk descriptions contained within this book.

Typeset by Simon and Sons
Printed and bound in India by Replika Press Pvt Ltd.

Contents

How to Use this Book

The walks in the book are ordered by distance, starting with the shortest. An information panel for each walk shows the distance, start point, a summary of route terrain and level of difficulty (easy/moderate/difficult), OS map(s) required, and suggested pubs/cafes at the start/end of walk or en route.

MAPS

There are eighty-four maps covering the 100 walks. Some of the walks are extensions of existing routes and the information panel for these walks will tell you the distance of the short and long versions of the walk. For those not wishing to undertake the longer versions of these walks, the 'short-cuts' are shown on the map in red. The routes marked on the maps are punctuated by a series of numbered waypoints. These relate to the same numbers shown in the walk description.

Start Points

The start of each walk is given as a postcode and also a six-figure grid reference number prefixed by two letters (which indicates the relevant square on the National Grid). More information on grid references is found on Ordnance Survey maps.

Parking

Many of the car parks suggested are public, but for some walks you will have to park on the roadside or in a lay-by. Please be considerate when leaving your car and do not block access roads or gates. Also, if parking in a pub car park for the duration of the walk, please try to avoid busy times.

COUNTRYSIDE CODE

- Consider the local community and other people enjoying the outdoors
- Leave gates and property as you find them and follow paths
- Leave no trace of your visit and take litter home
- Keep dogs under effective control
- Plan ahead and be prepared
- Follow advice and local signs

Walks Locator

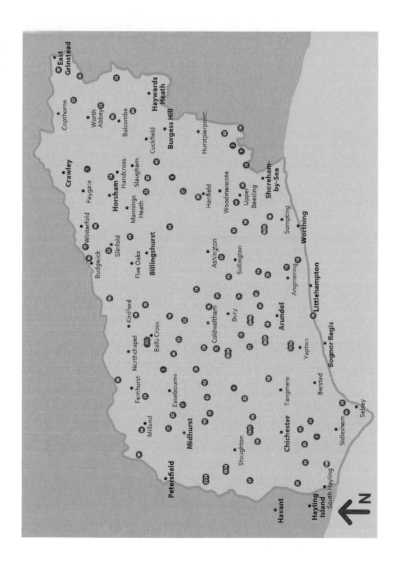

Buchan Country Park

START Buchan Country Park car park, RH11 9HQ, TQ245345

DISTANCE 1¾ miles (2.8km)

SUMMARY A family-friendly route through woodland and parkland along accessible paths

PARKING Large car park. Postcode: RH11 9HQ. To check car park opening times, visit: www.westsussex. gov.uk/leisure-recreation-and-community/places-to-visit-and-explore/buchan-country-park/

MAPS OS Explorer OL34; Landranger 187

WHERE TO EAT AND DRINK None en route; picnic area close to the end of the walk

Buchan Country Park offers a tranquil slice of countryside right on Crawley's doorstep and is perfect for a family walk.

1   Facing away from the car park entrance, walk past the visitor centre into Buchan Country Park. Cross the footbridge and once over the busy A-road, keep straight ahead walking towards Douster Pond. With the pond to your right continue straight ahead and once past the pond follow the tarmac path leading gently uphill through the trees. Ignore two turnings off to the right and then another path off to the left as you walk along this woodland stretch.

2   When you reach a fork go left (following the post signed with a red arrow). You soon emerge from the woods into an open wildflower meadow. Follow the path along the left-hand side of the meadow, which quickly takes you back into woodland and then winds its way through trees. When you reach a fork in the path go right and then shortly after at the next junction, go right again (you will see a golf course behind a fence on the right along here).

3   Follow this path as it takes you along the park boundary, ignoring any turnings off to the right. The path dips steeply down and as you reach the bottom, turn left (following the blue arrow). Walk through a small patch of heathland and past some pine trees then head back into

the woodland again. Cross a small footbridge and then at the crossroads go straight ahead, walking towards the pond. You will soon pass the 'dog dip' area on the left before the path takes you between Douster Pond to your right and Island Pond on the left.

4 Once over the water, bear right at the fork and follow the footpath along the edge of the pond up to a picnic area on the left. At the T-junction, turn right and retrace your steps past Douster Pond, across the road bridge, and back to the car park, where the walk began.

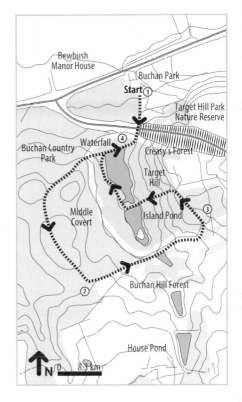

Points of interest

The two large ponds on this route were man-made by damming nearby Douster Brook. They were created as fishing ponds for the nineteenth-century landowner, Mr Phillipe Saillard, a French businessman who made his fortune selling playing cards and ostrich feathers for Victorian ladies' hats. Nowadays the ponds are still used for angling but are also home to a number of species of dragonfly, making them a Site of Special Scientific Interest.

Newtimber Hill

START Saddlescombe Farm (small car park opposite), BN45 7DE, TQ266120

DISTANCE 2¼ miles (3.6km)

SUMMARY A circular hilly route following footpaths and National Trust permissive paths around Newtimber Hill

PARKING Small free car park opposite the start point. Postcode: BN45 7DE

MAPS OS Explorer OL11; Landranger 198

WHERE TO EAT AND DRINK The Wildflour Cafe at Saddlescombe Farm (wildflourcafe.business.site – check website for opening times as the cafe is not open all year round)

A short but glorious walk offering outstanding views across West and East Sussex from the top of Newtimber Hill.

① From the car park, cross the road and follow the South Downs Way into Saddlescombe Farm and past some farm cottages. While owned by the National Trust with attractions open for visitors some of the time, Saddlescombe is still a working farm, as it has been for centuries.

② At a junction by a four-way fingerpost, leave the South Downs Way and turn left, walk a few paces to the fork, then go left again following the bridleway leading through the valley for approximately ¼ mile until you reach a gate.

③ Once through the gate make your way diagonally uphill. The views start to open up as you climb. This stretch contains the remains of Bronze Age cross dykes, ridges in the landscape thought to be prehistoric boundary markers. Continue straight ahead over the brow of the hill, then at a T-junction by a large oak tree with a gate to your right, turn left.

④ Follow the fairly indistinct path as it winds through gorse bushes and then alongside woodland. After approximately 300yds turn right onto a large clearing and walk a short distance enjoying the views as they open out ahead of you, before turning left. Follow the hillside path as it leads around Newtimber Hill, admiring the far-reaching views over the village of Poynings and surrounding countryside as you go.

5 Continue to follow the path around the flank of the hill for around ½ mile. The cattle-trodden path descends down to a gate leading back to Saddlescombe Farm. There are earthworks to your left on North Hill along this stretch.

6 Once back at the farm turn right and rejoin the South Downs Way, walking back to the road and the car park, the start and end point of the route.

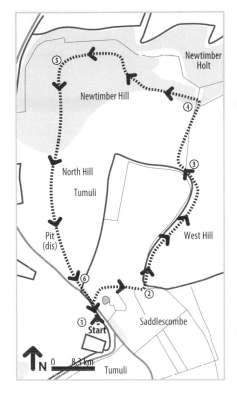

Points of interest

Saddlescombe has been a settlement for thousands of years and the National Trust information barn at Saddlescombe Farm displays artefacts showing human activity all the way back to the Stone Age. The farm itself has been in use in one form or another for more than 1,000 years, including being farmed by the Knights Templar during the thirteenth century. The oldest remaining farm buildings on the site date back to the early 1600s and include a well-preserved donkey wheel which was powered by a donkey to pull water from a well.

Chichester Marina and Birdham Pool

START Chichester Marina car park, PO20 7EJ, SU835010

DISTANCE 2½ miles (4km)

SUMMARY A circular route along accessible footpaths and country lanes

PARKING Free visitor car park at Chichester Marina. Postcode: PO20 7EJ

MAPS OS Explorer OL08; Landranger 197

WHERE TO EAT AND DRINK The Boat House Cafe (idealcollection. co.uk/venues/the-boathouse-cafe-chichester/)

A short, accessible route around Chichester Marina and Birdham Pool allowing everyone to enjoy this designated Area of Outstanding Natural Beauty.

1 From the car park, turn right and walk past the barrier into Chichester Marina. Follow the footpath along the road with the boats to your left until you arrive at the edge of Chichester Harbour.

2 Turn left here and walk with the open water to your right and the boats to your left. This path takes you across the lock and past the Boat House Cafe. When you reach the canal turn right and follow the path running alongside the houseboats to a footbridge across the water.

3 Cross the bridge and follow the path along an alley, ignoring a footpath turning to the right. Turn right at the end of the alleyway and go through a gate, then cross the road and walk straight ahead into Birdham Pool Marina.

4 Walk through Birdham Pool Marina, then follow the path as it bears left leading onto a lane. Ignore a footpath going off to the right and instead keep following the lane down to a church at the bottom of the road.

5 Once at the church, go left along the road and follow it for a short distance as it twists and turns before turning left again into Martins Lane (signed for the Salterns Way). Follow the quiet road, ignoring a right-hand footpath into a field when you reach a corner and another on the left leading behind houses back to Birdham Pool. Continue along the lane until you get to a private road on the right.

6 Go right and follow the signed footpath to the end of the road, then pass by a gate and cross the canal bridge leading back into Chichester Marina. Turn right and follow the footpath as it leads you back to the start point with the canal and houseboats on your right and the marina boats on your left as you walk.

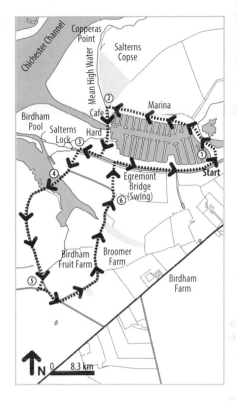

Points of interest

Birdham Pool Marina and Chichester Marina are thought to be among the oldest marinas in the UK. Birdham Pool has its origins in the 1930s when the marina was created out of the tidal mill pool of Birdham Mill, an eighteenth-century mill that was closed and sold off in 1935. The old mill is still standing and is now a listed building.

Meanwhile, nearby Chichester Marina was created in the 1960s and is also thought to be one of the oldest in the country.

Cowfold

START The Allmond Centre,
RH13 8BL, TQ214225

DISTANCE 2½ miles (4km)

SUMMARY An easy-going figure-
of-eight route along lanes and
footpaths; plenty of stiles

PARKING Free car park with
approximately twenty spaces.
Postcode: RH13 8BL

MAPS OS Explorer OL34;
Landranger 198

WHERE TO EAT AND DRINK The Hare
and Hounds pub is close to the start
and end of the walk (01403 865354)

A gentle walk along the quiet lanes, fields and farmland surrounding the village
of Cowfold.

1   With the Allmond Centre to your left and the children's playground
to your right, cross the playing field, then at the scout hut cross the main
road and turn left. Walk past some bungalows, ignoring the first footpath
to the right, and at the entrance for Eastlands House, go right.

Follow the public footpath along the drive and as you approach the
house, turn right walking towards the gate. Cross the stile and continue
straight ahead along the lane.

2   When you arrive at a junction where another lane joins from the right,
walk straight ahead and almost immediately turn left taking a footpath into
a field. Walk towards the next stile, then cross the field that has a small pond
over to the right. Climb the next stile and go over a small footbridge, then
continue straight ahead keeping the hedgerow to your left.

A metal bridge takes you over a stream, then continue straight ahead
to a gate and follow the path with a hedgerow to your right. At the end
of the path go through a gate into a meadow and follow the footpath
diagonally across. Turn right onto Moatfield Lane.

3   When you reach a house by Lower Barn Farm turn right to follow
a signed bridleway into a field. Cross the field and then a small stone
footbridge imprinted with horse footprints. Continue straight ahead
to a gate, then follow the narrow bridleway between hedgerows. After
approximately 300yds, climb a stile on your right.

④ Follow the public footpath across the field and then between two oak trees. Turn left and over a stile, then right onto a track leading up to a metal gate.

Follow the track past Baldwins Farm and onto the lane. Keep straight ahead, ignoring any turnings off to the left or right. The lane dips then rises again where it crosses Cowfold Stream.

⑤ When you arrive at a junction with another lane, go left and head towards woodland (this is the junction you passed early on in the walk). Follow the lane past some allotments, then at the pub turn right. Follow the road up to a roundabout then turn right again and head back to the start point.

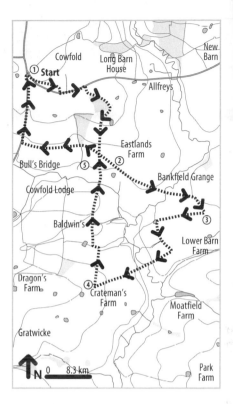

Points of interest

The Cowfold Stream, which you encounter several times on this walk, is a tributary of the River Adur and also acts as a boundary between Cowfold and the nearby parish of Shermanbury.

START The Hollist Arms, The Street, Lodsworth, GU28 9BZ, SU927231

DISTANCE 3 miles (4.8km)

SUMMARY An easy walk following footpaths, bridleways and lanes; much of the route is through woodland so it can be muddy

PARKING Roadside parking near the pub. Postcode: GU28 9BZ

MAPS OS Explorer OL33; Landranger 197

WHERE TO EAT AND DRINK The Hollist Arms is at the start and end point (thehollistarms.com); the Halfway Bridge is also passed on this route (halfwaybridge.co.uk)

A walk through the woodlands and countryside surrounding the village of Lodsworth in an area of outstanding natural beauty.

1   With the pub to your right follow The Street down the hill through the village. When you get to Church Lane turn left into it and walk down to the church. Once at the church gate go right following the bridleway past cottages. When you reach the corner ignore a footpath straight ahead and instead follow the bridleway to the left and then the right. Head through the trees and then bear right, following the bridleway between hedgerows. Remain straight ahead on this bridleway until you arrive at a lane.

2   Turn left at the lane and walk past the Halfway Bridge pub to your right. Continue along the lane until you reach a fairly wide signed footpath on the left leading between hedgerows. Take this path and follow it gently uphill. At a three-way fingerpost by a stile go left and climb another stile heading into woods. The River Lod runs to your left down a steep valley. Keep straight ahead until you reach a junction with a bridleway then bear right, taking the bridleway uphill to reach a lane.

3   At River Lane go left. Ignore a footpath on the right leading up steps and instead continue straight ahead following the lane downhill. Shortly after take a narrow footpath on the left down three steps. The footpath leads you back into woodland. Follow the obvious footpath through the woods (can be muddy) and when the path forks, bear right and head downhill.

④ At the bottom of the hill you meet a junction with a bridleway. Take the bridleway right and cross a bridge. Once across continue straight ahead following the bridleway through the middle of the field. Go though the gate on the opposite side and turn right onto the footpath. Follow the footpath towards the trees (ignoring a right turning through a gate). The path leads across footbridges and back into woodland.

⑤ When the path forks, go left. You soon cross another footbridge over a stream then emerge from the woods. Head uphill to reach the village lane. At The Street turn left and head back to the pub by the start point.

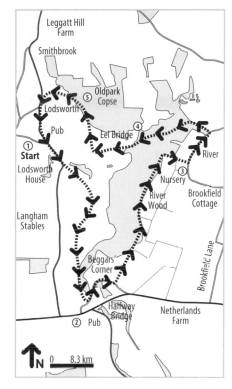

Points of interest

E. H. Shepard, the illustrator of *Winnie the Pooh* and *The Wind in the Willows* lived in Lodsworth towards the end of his life. His house has a commemorative blue plaque and his grave can be found in the churchyard.

East Dean

START Main Road, East Dean, PO18 0JG, SU905131

DISTANCE 3 miles (5km)

SUMMARY An easy circular walk on bridleways and footpaths

PARKING Roadside parking in East Dean. Postcode: PO18 0JG

MAPS OS Explorer OL10; Landranger 197

WHERE TO EAT AND DRINK The Star and Garter pub is close to the start and end point of the walk (thestarandgarter.co.uk/)

A short, family-friendly circular walk starting from the quaint village of East Dean.

1 From East Dean village follow the main road with the pub to your right passing All Saints church on the left as you go. Once past the church continue past a row of houses on the left until you come to a corner with a lay-by. Go left here, leaving the road and following the wide public way leading gently uphill. After a short distance you will see a footpath going off to the left, ignore this and continue straight ahead.

2 When you reach a three-way fingerpost by a large Charlton Forest Forestry Commission sign, turn left and follow the bridleway through the woods. The views soon open out across the valley. Walk for approximately ¼ mile and then at the next junction by a three-way fingerpost turn right.

3 Follow the bridleway straight ahead for another ¼ mile until it turns sharp left (signed). The bridleway then leads steeply downhill towards farm buildings. To avoid such a steep descent you can follow a track straight ahead which leads you down more gently to reach the public way. At the bottom go left again following the public way for around ½ mile to reach some large farm buildings.

4 At the farm ignore the first right-hand sign for a bridleway and instead continue for a few paces and take the next right turning for a footpath. This leads you between two barns and to a gated field. At the gate turn left and follow the footpath through a kissing gate and into the field.

5 The footpath skirts the lower edge of the field before heading into woodland. Follow the path as it leads up through the woods until it meets a bridleway at a field.

6 Follow the bridleway along the lower edge of the field and then down to a gate. There is a well-placed bench here with views to the twelfth-century All Saints church and surrounding countryside. After you've stopped to take in the views, go through the gate and then at the T-junction go left and walk down to the lane. Turn right at the lane and follow it back to the main road and East Dean village.

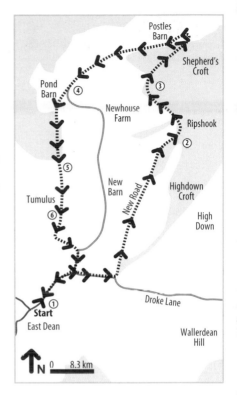

Points of interest

The River Lavant which flows down to Chichester Harbour rises in the village of East Dean with the village pond as its source. The Lavant is often dry but in 1994 it burst its banks, flooding Chichester and the surrounding areas.

Ebernoe Common

START Ebernoe Holy Trinity church, GU28 9LD, SU974278

DISTANCE 3 miles (4.7km) or 4¾ miles (7.6km)

SUMMARY Two walks mainly along woodland footpaths and some lanes; can be muddy

PARKING Free car park at the start point. Postcode: GU28 9LD

MAPS OS Explorer OL33; Landranger 197

WHERE TO EAT AND DRINK The Stag Inn, Balls Cross is passed on the longer route (staginnballscross.co.uk)

Two peaceful routes through ancient woodland, which is full of wildflowers during the spring.

1 With the church and car park to your right follow the public way down to a cattle grid and enter Ebernoe Common Nature Reserve. Take the first signed footpath right and walk for approximately 200yds to where the path forks.

2 Go left and follow the footpath through the woodland for around ½ mile until you reach a gate.
    For the shorter route, turn right here and then follow instructions from point 6.

3 For the longer route go through the gate and follow the drive to a T-junction, then turn right and walk to a road.

4 Turn right and follow the lane in the direction of Balls Cross for ¼ mile until you meet another road. Go right here walking past the Stag Inn and continue on for just over ½ mile.

5 Take a public footpath right and follow it into Langhurst Common. Follow the woodland footpath for ¾ mile as it takes you past grand old trees and crosses numerous footbridges. When you arrive back at the gate you encountered earlier on the walk go through and turn left.

6 Walk a short distance to a fingerpost and go left (or right on shorter route). Walk straight ahead along this woodland footpath for just under ½ mile to reach a footpath turning on the right.

7 Turn right and follow the path across a stream and then round to the left. Continue for ⅓ mile to the next junction.

8 Turn left to follow the footpath through a gate. The path descends to a footbridge, then climbs up steps and crosses another bridge. Cross a field, then turn right at the T-junction and continue to a road.

9 Turn right and walk to where the road bends then follow the signed footpath into the woodland. Go left and walk alongside a field for around 100yds until the footpath forks. Go right and follow the path straight ahead through the woods ignoring any turnings off either side. This leads you down to a stream and then up to a stile. Cross the stile into the field, then walk straight ahead to a gate.

10 Turn left and walk a short distance to another fingerpost where you continue straight ahead. This final part of the walk retraces your earlier steps. Walk up to the T-junction, turn left and then follow the public way back up to Ebernoe church.

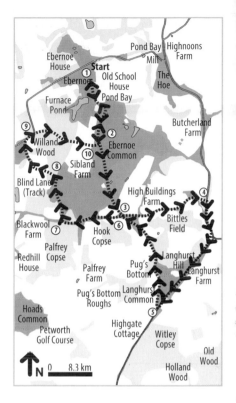

Points of interest

Ebernoe Common is ancient wood pasture that was used by Commoners to graze pigs and cattle until the mid twentieth century.

Devil's Dyke

START Devil's Dyke car park,
BN1 8YJ, TQ267096

DISTANCE 3 miles (5km)

SUMMARY A short but moderate
route along footpaths and bridleways

PARKING Large (but can be
busy) car park at the start
point. Postcode: BN1 8YJ

MAPS OS Explorer OL11;
Landranger 198

WHERE TO EAT AND DRINK Devil's
Dyke pub next to the start point
or Royal Oak in Poynings, midway
through the walk (vintageinn.
co.uk/restaurants/south-east/
thedevilsdykebrighton; www.
royaloakpoynings.pub)

A circular route with plenty of ups and downs and breathtaking views over the
Devil's Dyke valley.

①   Start with the pub to your right and walk right the way around it to
join the footpath leading out of the car park heading towards the valley.
Follow the footpath for just over ¼ mile taking in the views. Ignore a left
turn down to a stile and footpath and instead continue straight ahead. The
path soon begins to head steeply downhill and arrives at a T-junction –
go left.

②   Follow the bridleway downhill (ignore a left turning). The path leads
through a gate into woodland. Ignore a left turn as you walk through the
woods and continue on. At the next three-way fingerpost go right and
follow the bridleway through fields to the nearby village of Poynings.

③   You emerge in the village opposite Dyke Farm House. Turn right
and walk past the Royal Oak, looking out for a right-hand footpath by a
garage.

④   Follow the footpath past the garage and into a field and then soon
go left over a stile. The path crosses a footbridge by a pond and then
runs alongside a field before heading into woodland. When you reach a
T-junction go right taking the bridleway downhill.

⑤   At a three-way fingerpost continue in the same direction along the
bridleway. When you reach a gate go back into the valley and take the left-
hand path uphill. When the path forks go left again, heading steeply up.

At the top, turn left and climb the ladder stile entering a field. Follow the path towards Saddlescombe Farm.

6 Turn right at the road and walk through a small car park. Take the South Downs Way from the top of the car park heading uphill. At the top of the hill by a three-way fingerpost go right remaining on the South Downs Way. At the next crossroads continue straight ahead along the South Downs Way, and then the same at the next junction. The pub at Devil's Dyke car park can now be seen over the valley to your right.

7 At the road leave the South Downs Way and turn right walking along the verge. Ignore a right bridleway and continue along the road walking back towards the pub.

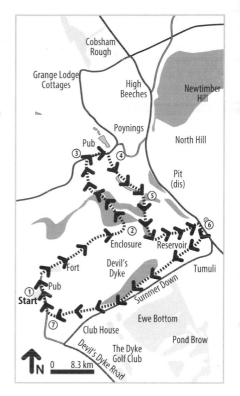

Points of interest

Devil's Dyke is the longest, deepest and widest 'dry valley' in the UK. According to legend it earned its name because the Devil became angry with people of the Weald turning to Christianity, and so carved the dyke in order to flood their villages.

Steyning

START Steyning long stay car park, BN44 3XZ, TQ178111

DISTANCE 3 miles (4.5km)

SUMMARY A moderate walk on footpaths, bridleways and lanes; one fairly steep climb up to the South Downs

PARKING Large pay and display car park. Postcode: BN44 3XZ

MAPS OS Explorer OL11; Landranger 198

WHERE TO EAT AND DRINK Plenty of choice of eateries in Steyning

A hike up to Steyning Coombe, where you can enjoy panoramic views over the rooftops of Steyning village and the countryside beyond.

1   From the south-western corner of the car park take an alleyway leading along School Lane, then turn right into Church Street. At the T-junction with the high street turn right and follow it until you see a set of stone steps signed for the Downs footpath on your left. Climb the steps and turn right once you reach the top, walking for approximately 100yds until you see a signpost for a footpath.

2   Leave the road here and follow the public footpath uphill towards Steyning Coombe. When you reach a gate continue straight ahead uphill, passing an information board and heading towards a well-placed bench at the top of the hill.

3   After stopping at the bench to admire the stunning views, go right and pass through a gate into some woodland. Turn right again following the track downhill for a short distance and then fork right. You will soon arrive at a field. Follow the bridleway along the edge of the field down to a metal gate and then turn right onto Mouse Lane.

4   Follow the quiet lane for approximately ¼ mile. There is a poem carved into a stone plaque along this stretch by First World War poet, John Stanley Purvis, expressing his love for the lane and the area. Towards the end of Mouse Lane you will also pass some very old cottages, which used to be used as a workhouse for the poor and destitute. When you reach the main road, bear right and walk back in the direction of the high street. When you reach Tanyard Lane, turn left and follow it towards the church.

⑤ At the T-junction by Shooting Field, cross the road and walk through the churchyard of the eleventh-century church of St Andrews. Once you've made your way through the churchyard (and popped into the old church for a look around), cross the road and return to the car park, where the walk begins and ends.

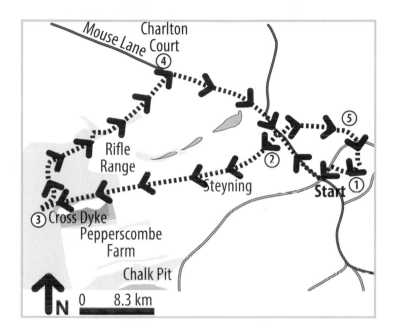

Petworth – Shimmings Valley

START Petworth main town centre
car park, GU28 0AP, SU976215

DISTANCE 3 miles (5km)

SUMMARY A short, moderate
walk along footpaths and lanes

PARKING Pay and display car park
(free on Sundays). Postcode: GU28 0AP

MAPS OS Explorer OL33;
Landranger 197

WHERE TO EAT AND DRINK
The Black Horse Inn in Byworth
(blackhorsebyworth.co.uk) is a short
detour midway through the walk

A beautiful circular walk between Petworth town centre and the hamlet of
Byworth, with fantastic views over the Shimmings Valley.

① From the car park take the alleyway leading to the market square.
Continue straight ahead towards the church, soon following the cobbles
of Lombard Street to reach the main road. Go right, then take the second
right into Barton Lane following it down past a churchyard to join a
footpath through gates.

② Follow the footpath downhill to a bridge over a stream, then continue
straight ahead. When you reach a three-way fingerpost signed for the
Serpent Trail remain straight ahead keeping the hedgerow to your left to
reach a kissing gate. Follow the path as it curves to the left passing a small
copse. Once under the pylon bear left heading towards a kissing gate. The
views are glorious along this stretch!

③ Follow the footpath through the gate and into the trees. Head steadily
up to reach Brinsole Heath, then at the broad path go right. When you
arrive at a fork in the path by a metal gate bear right, continuing for a
short distance to a three-way fingerpost.

④ Turn sharp right here, walking towards a pair of grand stone gates.
At the gates turn left and follow the path down past farm buildings. When
the track swings to the right, keep straight ahead, taking the footpath
through a kissing gate leading between fenced-in fields.

⑤ At the road turn right, then cross with care and take the footpath
opposite over a stile. Follow the indistinct path diagonally across the field

to the bottom corner, then pass through two gates to reach a lane. Turn right and walk to a cottage (with a Hovis sign) by a red phone box. Go left here and head down to a kissing gate and past a pond. Cross a stile and bear left along the bottom edge of a paddock to reach another stile. Once over, turn left and head down to cross a stream before arriving at a T-junction.

6 Go right and when the path soon forks, go left. At the top of the hill continue straight ahead following the path as it winds around a farm before passing allotments and arriving at a lane.

7 Go right, to reach Rosemary Lane, then turn left. At the end of this road follow the alley back to the car park.

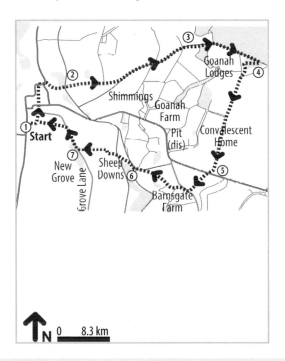

Points of interest

While most famous for the grand Petworth House, the small market town is itself an architectural treasure trove well worth exploring, with many historic buildings dating back hundreds of years.

Fulking

START Shepherd and Dog
pub, BN5 9LU, TQ247114

DISTANCE 3 miles (5km)

SUMMARY A moderate walk along
footpaths, bridleways, tracks
and a short stretch of road; very
steep climb early on in the walk

PARKING Free roadside parking
in Fulking village by the pub
(can get busy, especially at
weekends). Postcode: BN5 9LU

MAPS OS Explorer OL11;
Landranger 198

WHERE TO EAT AND DRINK The
Shepherd and Dog pub is at the
start and end point of the walk
(shepherdanddogpub.co.uk)

A steep climb takes you up from the pretty village of Fulking to the South Downs
Way with fantastic views out to sea.

① Start by facing the Shepherd and Dog and take the signed bridleway
to the left of the pub. Shortly after turn right onto a public footpath up
some steps leading you behind the pub garden. Climb a stile and follow
the steps uphill.

② When you reach the Fulking escarpment, keep straight ahead,
continuing to climb steeply. At the top you will reach a four-way
fingerpost. Continue straight ahead again. Go through a gate and follow
the public footpath up towards the hilltop.

③ At the next junction, go left and follow the main track round towards
the ruins of an old building and a trig point. Once past the trig point head to
a stile, climb over and turn right onto the lane (Devil's Dyke is to your left). After
a short distance turn right, passing through the gate to follow the bridleway
ahead. You are now on the South Downs Way and on a clear day you get
glorious sea views along this stretch over nearby Brighton and Shoreham.

④ At the gate continue straight ahead following the South Downs Way
for just under 1 mile. Keep your eyes peeled for the remains of the Fulking
Isolation Hospital along here to your left in amongst a clump of trees. Just
past the remnants of the old hospital, ignore a turning to your right, and
continue ahead until you reach a crossroads.

5 Turn right here onto a public footpath and head down past a pylon before turning off the footpath and following the wide bostal track as it winds downhill. At a bend in the track you will see an old Victorian lime kiln on your left.

6 When you get to a fence leave the bostal track and turn right onto a footpath. Continue straight ahead along this path with the fence to your left ignoring any turnings off. The path dips down at a clearing by a trough and continues ahead becoming narrower. Follow the path around the hill to reach the steps you came up earlier at point 2. Turn left here and head downhill, back towards the pub.

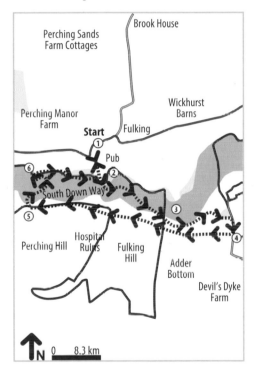

Points of interest

Fulking Isolation Hospital, known as Fulking Grange, was built in 1901 and used to isolate patients suffering from infectious diseases such as smallpox. The hospital was closed after it was requisitioned for military use in 1940 and now lies in ruins.

Compton

START The Square, Compton,
PO18 9HA, SU776148

DISTANCE 3 miles (4.6km)
or 5 miles (8km)

SUMMARY Two moderate walks
following footpaths, bridleways lanes,
and short sections of roadside walking

PARKING Small parking area at
the start. Postcode: PO18 9HA

MAPS OS Explorer OL08;
Landranger 197

WHERE TO EAT AND DRINK
The Coach and Horses is
at the start and end point
(coachandhorsescompton.co.uk)

Two beautiful downland walks from the village of Compton in the South Downs
National Park.

①   From the parking area, with the pub to your right, walk up School
Lane and take the public way uphill. You will shortly arrive at a junction,
bear right and continue uphill along the bridleway. At the T-junction go
right and head downhill.

②   When the bridleway meets a lane turn right towards West Marden.
At the main road, cross over, and follow the lane opposite.

③   Walk past the pub (Victoria Inn) and continue straight ahead
ignoring a turning on the left. When the road bends round to the left walk
straight ahead, taking a bridleway uphill through trees. The path wiggles
and climbs to a T-junction.

④   At the T-junction go right and follow the bridleway a short distance
to where the path forks. Go right and walk to a three-way fingerpost.

⑤a. For the shorter route take the right footpath to reach a metal kissing
gate. Follow the footpath to the left as the views open out. The path winds
down through the meadow and then rises up again following a track to a
field with a four-way footpath junction.

⑥a. Take the middle footpath leading diagonally left through the field
heading back to Compton. On the opposite side go through the metal gate
and continue straight ahead downhill, then through the next gate. You soon
arrive at another field. Follow the path diagonally across the field to a line of

trees. Continue diagonally across the next field towards houses. When you get to the other side descend the steps and turn left, following the road back to the start point.

5   For the longer route go left. Follow the bridleway for around ½ mile as it winds its way to reach woodland.

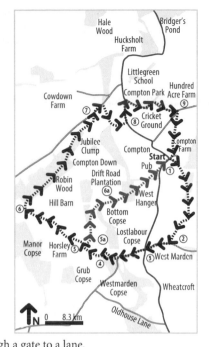

6   As you enter the woodland the path splits. Ignore the left footpath turning and take the bridleway ahead. When the path soon forks, go right. Follow the bridleway straight ahead, ignoring a left and right footpath turning as you walk through the woodland for around ½ mile. At a clearing the bridleway swings left and starts to head downhill and on to a gate where views open out. Continue with trees to your right to another gate. Once through continue on to the next gate, entering a meadow. Go left and walk towards a fence, then through a gate to a lane.

7   Turn right and follow the road to reach a right footpath turning. Follow the path down through the same meadow heading back towards woodland to a kissing gate. Continue on the footpath to reach a road.

8   Turn left and follow the roadside verge for around 270yds. When you reach a lane, turn right. Follow the wiggly lane for ½ mile to a road junction. Here turn right them immediately take a footpath on the left leading across a field.

9   Cross the field diagonally to a meadow. Follow the footpath to a kissing gate on the other side of the meadow then follow a track past buildings to a lane. Turn right and follow the lane back to the start point.

Points of interest

Nearby Uppark can be seen from various points along the routes. The grand seventeenth-century mansion house is now a National Trust property.

START Highdown Gardens,
Worthing, BN12 6FB, TQ099037

DISTANCE 3¼ miles (5.3km)

SUMMARY An easy walk
following footpaths, bridleways
and one stretch of road

PARKING Free car park at the
start point. Postcode: BN12 6FB

MAPS OS Explorer OL10;
Landranger 198

WHERE TO EAT AND DRINK
Tearoom and restaurant at Highdown
Gardens (www.brunningandprice.
co.uk/highdown/tearoom/

This stroll around Highdown Hill offers beautiful views and a peaceful historic garden to visit.

1   Turn left out of the car park and head uphill along the road. Once at the top, with Highdown Gardens to your left, take the exit out of the top right corner of the car park and head left following the footpath as it curves around and leads uphill to the Miller's Tomb. Walk past the tomb and through a gate then continue straight ahead across the downs enjoying the views as you walk.

2   When you reach a four-way fingerpost continue straight ahead. This leads you past earthworks on the right. Keep walking for around ¼ mile to reach a gate by a crossroads.

3   Go through the gate and walk through the centre of the field towards the mill (the path is fenced in on either side). The path veers to the right and then turns sharp left. Walk past the mill and at the end of the path turn left.

4   Follow the bridleway, which begins to lead gently uphill and then slopes down until you reach a junction of footpaths and bridleways with a set of steps to the left.

5   Ignore the left turning and instead continue on the bridleway, turning left after a few paces. The path heads up and arrives at a fork, bear right here remaining on the lower path leading past paddocks. Stick to the main chalky path ignoring a path forking off to the right towards the end of the paddocks and follow it as it winds its way uphill.

6 The path soon forks again; bear left to follow the bridleway up towards the four-way fingerpost you passed earlier at point 2 of the walk. This time go straight ahead.

7 When you reach the hedgerow turn right and follow the bridleway back down to the Highdown Gardens car park. After popping into Highdown Gardens (highly recommended), head back downhill to the start and end point of the walk.

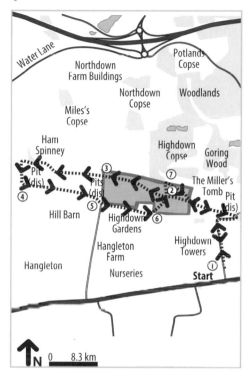

Points of interest

Highdown Gardens is free to visitors and well worth a look on the way past. The peaceful chalk gardens were created at the beginning of the twentieth century by an aristocratic family, the Sterns, who hired plant hunters to collect seeds and cuttings from around the world. The garden was donated to Worthing Council by Lady Sybil Stern after her husband Sir Frederick Stern's death in 1968, as she wanted to preserve them for the benefit of the public.

The Mens

START The Mens Sussex Wildlife Trust car park, RH14 0HR, TQ023236

DISTANCE 3¼ miles (5.2km)

SUMMARY A circular woodland walk along footpaths, bridleways and quiet lanes; can be muddy

PARKING Free Sussex Wildlife Trust car park (small). Postcode: RH14 0HR

MAPS OS Explorer OL34; Landranger 197

WHERE TO EAT AND DRINK None en route; the Half Moon Pub is in the nearby village of Kirdford (halfmoonkirdford.co.uk)

A tranquil walk through the ancient woodland of The Mens Sussex Wildlife Trust Nature Reserve.

1   Leave the car park via the quiet road and turn right. After approximately 10yds take the unmarked trail on the opposite side and follow the track as it winds through the ancient woodland. Cross a footbridge made from railway sleepers over a small brook and continue to follow the trail through the woodland until you arrive at a T-junction (bluebells here in spring).

2   At the T-junction turn right onto the bridleway and follow it past a house on the right ignoring any turnings off the main path. Pass a white house on your left before the bridleway narrows and continues through woodland, then leads down to another footbridge. Once over the brook, bear right and continue along the bridleway, which starts to climb uphill. Remain on this bridleway until you reach a quiet lane.

3   At the lane turn left and follow it to the end where it reaches Fittleworth Road. Turn right here and continue along the road as it weaves around to the right until you reach a right-hand turning for Brick Kiln Common. Go right here and follow the lane past some houses tucked away in the woodland.

4   At a sign for Kiln Cottage by a three-way footpath sign, turn right onto a gravel path. Follow the footpath, passing the house on your right, as it leads back into woodland and then downhill. Cross a small

footbridge over a stream and then follow the footpath as it climbs back up to a gate. Go through the gate, then walk a couple of paces and turn right. Follow the footpath along the right-hand edge of a few fields before you arrive at another gate.

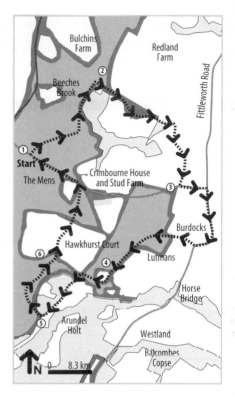

5 Go through the gate and turn right. Follow the footpath straight ahead to a T-junction with a bridleway. Turn right and follow the bridleway down until you reach a quiet lane. Turn left and head downhill, crossing a stream, before heading back up again to Hawkhurst Court.

6 Follow the bridleway all the way through Hawkhurst Court and continue straight ahead until you reach another lane. Turn left here and follow it back up to the Sussex Wildlife Trust car park.

Points of interest

The Mens Sussex Wildlife Trust site is home to rare purple emperor butterflies as well as wildflowers such as violet helleborine and yellow archangel. Much of the ancient woodland is carpeted in bluebells in late spring.

START Midhurst, North Street car park, GU29 9DW, SU886218

DISTANCE 3¼ miles (5.2km)

SUMMARY An easy route along the River Rother and through Midhurst

PARKING Large pay and display car park at start and end of walk. Postcode: GU29 9DW

MAPS OS Explorer OL33; Landranger 197

WHERE TO EAT AND DRINK The Half Moon pub is close to the end of the walk

This route takes you past the ruins of a Tudor manor house, along the meandering river Rother and through National Trust parkland, before winding its way back through the pretty market town of Midhurst.

① The walk begins with a quick glimpse at the ruins of Cowdray House and the surrounding estate. Leave the car park via the main entrance and follow the signed footpath towards the ruins. At Cowdray House turn left. Shortly after the path forks, bear left to follow the lane. At the road turn left, then immediately cross the road and walk over the bridge with a weir to your right. Once across take the right-hand footpath signed for Rother Walk.

② Follow the footpath as it winds through scrubby woodland and along the water's edge. When you come to a fork, bear right and continue along the riverside. The landscape soon opens out. After approximately ½ mile you will reach a boardwalk, which takes you over soggy ground.

③ Cross the boardwalk and walk up to a field, then turn right. When you reach the far corner of the field go right and follow the path down into the next field. Continue walking until you reach a National Trust sign for Woolbeding parkland. Go through the gate and follow the path diagonally up through the field. There is a folly to your left which is part of Woolbeding House, a grand Georgian building you can see over to your right that wouldn't seem out of place in a Jane Austen novel.

④ At the top of the field, pass through the next gate into a patch of woodland.

The landscape soon opens up again with the path leading downhill through the parkland to another gate. At the gate go left, leaving the signed Rother Walk and following the public footpath along the bottom edge of the field. This footpath leads to a gate and then a stile. Once over the stile go right, crossing a small footbridge, then continue along the path to the road.

⑤ At the road turn left, walking towards the Half Moon pub where you turn left again and follow the lane all the way to Midhurst town centre. At the high street go left. This leads you along the main shopping street and back to the car park.

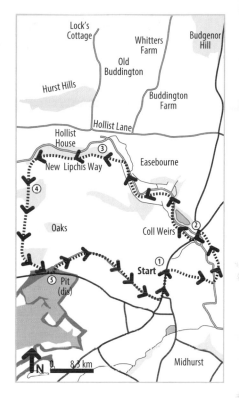

Points of interest

Cowdray House now lies in ruins after a fire swept through it in 1793, but in its heyday it played host to Tudor kings and queens such as Henry VIII and Elizabeth I. Another famous resident was Guy Fawkes, who reputedly once worked there.

START Pulborough town centre car park, RH20 2BF, TQ053185

DISTANCE 3¼ miles (5.25km)

SUMMARY An easy walk along footpaths and one stretch of road; much of this route is through water meadows so best to walk it during dry months

PARKING Pay and display car park at the start point. Postcode: RH20 2BF

MAPS OS Explorer OL10; Landranger 197

WHERE TO EAT AND DRINK The Little Bean Cafe is close to the start point (littlebeancafe.co.uk)

A peaceful walk through the water meadows of the Arun valley, just south of Pulborough.

1️⃣ From the town centre car park, walk back up to the main road and turn right. Follow the main road through Pulborough for just over ½ mile to reach a farm and a footpath turning on the right.

2️⃣ Take this turning and follow a surfaced path to begin with, then bear left and follow the footpath as it follows the course of a stream. Climb a stile into a field and walk across to the riverbank, then walk with the water to your left to reach a bridge.

3️⃣ Cross the bridge and follow the footpath towards a gate and a stile, then once over the stile, continue following the footpath for just over ⅓ mile with water meadows to your right. There are more stiles to climb along this stretch. Just after passing a cottage, the footpath bears left through a kissing gate. Continue to some steps, then turn right and shortly after turn left through another kissing gate, entering a field. Follow the footpath as it skirts the field and enters another. Walk past a farm on the right before arriving at the tiny village of Wiggonholt.

4️⃣ When you arrive at Wiggonholt parish church follow the lane to a signed footpath by a gate. Turn right through the gate and follow the broad path past the church ignoring a turning on the left. This stretch leads you through a section of the RSPB Pulborough Brookes Nature Reserve. Continue to follow the clearly signed footpath through gates to reach a field. Cross the field and then go through another gate before heading downhill to the banks of the River Arun.

5 At the Arun, go right and follow the riverside path for nearly ½ mile enjoying the views as you walk along the riverbank. Cross a footbridge, then when the path forks, bear diagonally left, walking back towards the houses. When you arrive at a cottage, go through a gate and follow the road to a set of steps on the right-hand side. Climb these to arrive back at the start point.

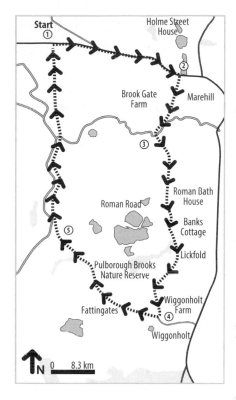

Points of interest

Wiggonholt parish church dates back to the twelfth century. The tiny church remains much in its original form.

Pulborough Brooks Nature Reserve: This RSPB reserve is home to many wildfowl and wetland bird species such as lapwing and wigeon. Nightingales, peregrine falcons and barn owls are also regular visitors to the site.

Cocking

START Cocking Hill car park, GU29 0HT, SU875166

DISTANCE 3¼ miles (5.2km)

SUMMARY A circular route on bridleways and restricted byways

PARKING Cocking Hill car park. Postcode: GU29 0HT

MAPS OS Explorer OL08; Landranger 197

WHERE TO EAT AND DRINK The Flint Barn Cafe is close to the start and end of the walk (flintbarncafe.co.uk)

A glorious circular route through woodland and open downland with wonderful views from the South Downs Way.

1   From the car park join the South Downs Way and turn left heading towards the Flint Barn Cafe. Walk past the cafe and continue straight ahead past farm buildings. The South Downs Way follows the lane and leads uphill for approximately ¾ mile.

2   When you arrive at a crossroads by a large chalk boulder, leave the South Downs Way and take the grassy bridleway forking off to the left. After around ¼ mile a bridleway turns off to the right. Ignore this turning and continue straight ahead.

3   After approximately 200yds you will arrive at another junction by another large boulder. Take the path on the right here and head towards the trees, then at the next junction shortly after go right again.

4   When you arrive back at the South Downs Way go straight ahead at the crossroads and follow the restricted byway leading gently downhill into the woods. The path soon begins to head more steeply down.
    Ignore a gate into access land on the left and continue to follow the chalky path downhill enjoying the views when they open out.

5   At the bottom of the hill, ignore a bridleway on the left and continue straight ahead following the byway as it winds through trees and then follows a grassy track between hedges.

6   When you arrive at a T-junction go right. The path soon swings left and heads downhill past a house and barn. At the bottom of the hill turn left again. Ignore a bridleway turning off to the right and instead continue ahead along the byway past the buildings. When the path forks shortly after, take the restricted byway signed for the South Downs Way leading up into the trees. This leads back up to the Flint Barn Cafe. Turn left to return to the car park.

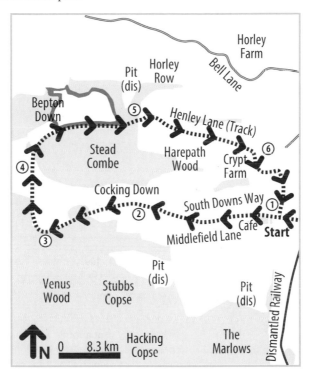

Points of interest

The large boulders seen on this walk are part of a collection of fourteen chalk sculptures placed in the landscape to form a 5-mile trail between Cocking and West Dean. They were created by Andy Goldsworthy in 2002 and the idea was for the bright white chalk boulders to create a moonlit path through the countryside. The work is ever evolving with the stones being left to weather in the landscape. They have also been used as part of a scientific study examining how quickly chalk disintegrates.

East Grinstead

START King Street car park, RH19 3DJ, TQ394382

DISTANCE 3½ miles (5.6km)

SUMMARY An easy urban walk following roads and footpaths

PARKING King Street car park. Postcode: RH19 3DJ

MAPS OS Explorer OL135; Landranger 187

WHERE TO EAT AND DRINK Plenty of places to eat and drink in East Grinstead

An urban and woodland walk through East Grinstead, exploring the sites and history of the town.

1   From the car park turn right heading past the public toilets. Just before you reach London Road, turn left into Institute Walk running along an alley. When you get to the road take the path opposite leading straight ahead. This takes you past a car park to reach Church Lane. Turn right into Church Lane, go straight ahead for 100m, and when you get to St Swithun's church entrance, follow the path through the churchyard to the high street.

2   At the high street turn left. Walk past Sackville College and go left into College Lane. Follow College Lane over the road bridge, then just after crossing Estcots Drive, take the path ahead leading into East Court, ignoring the sign for the Sussex Border path.

3   Follow the path through the grounds of East Court, once a grand eighteenth-century house and now council buildings. Walk past a children's playground and then bear left when the road forks. Continue to a set of steps, then cross a drive and shortly reach the main road.

4   At the main road (Holtye Road) turn right. Walk a short distance and then take the first right into Lynton Park Avenue. Follow the residential road all the way to the end. When you reach a T-junction with Lancaster Drive, go right and then follow it to Fulmar Drive. Take this road heading uphill to reach Stirling Way on the left. Turn into Stirling Way and go through the gate.

5 Follow the path through the trees leading into woodland. Ignore any turnings off either side and continue on for just over ¼ mile where the path heads down to a stream. Cross the bridge and continue along the path to reach a junction with a footpath where you turn left. Follow the path past a pond and then take a right-hand path before the playing field. When you arrive at the road go right and shortly after take a left-hand path heading uphill and past the mansion house.

6 Once past East Court Mansion, turn right and follow the path back up to the children's playground you passed earlier (it's worth a quick detour here to visit the War Memorial Garden). Once back at the playground turn left and follow the path out of East Court grounds and back to the road. At College Lane go straight on, then just before the road bridge, turn right into Sandy Lane. Follow the narrow lane to the end and then turn left to cross the bridge into Christopher Road and return to the car park.

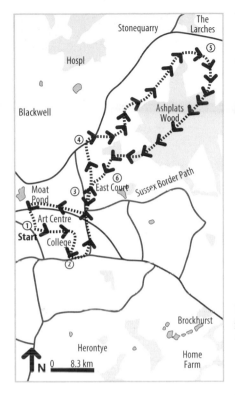

Points of interest

Sackville College is a Jacobean almshouse built out of sandstone and founded in 1609. Today it is still used as accommodation for the elderly.

Madehurst

START Stammers Lane,
BN18 0NT, SU979111

DISTANCE 3½ miles (5.6km)

SUMMARY An easy circular route
along forest and farmland bridleways

PARKING Limited roadside
parking at the end of Stammers
Lane. Postcode: BN18 0NT

MAPS OS Explorer OL10;
Landranger 197

**WHERE TO EAT AND
DRINK** None en route

A circular walk through the countryside surrounding Madehurst with fantastic
views over the South Downs and out to sea.

[1] The walk begins on Stammers Lane in the tiny village of Madehurst.
From the end of the lane, follow the bridleway straight ahead climbing
gently uphill. At a T-junction go left and walk along the field's edge. Once
across the field continue straight ahead through the valley with trees
either side. At the fork go left through the woods and then when you
reach a field, turn right. Walk for around 20yds and then take the next left
footpath, heading back into woodland.

[2] When you arrive at a T-junction soon after, turn right and follow this
bridleway straight ahead for ½ mile, ignoring any turnings off the path as
you go (including two bridleways on the left).

[3] At the T-junction (by Gumber Corner) turn right and follow the
wide bridleway for approximately ¼ mile. This stretch provides wide-
reaching views over the surrounding countryside and out to the coast
a few miles away. Ignore any turnings on the left until you reach a
crossroads beside a chunky wooden bench carved out of a tree trunk.

[4] With the tree trunk bench to your left continue straight ahead,
following the bridleway with trees to your right. Neolithic artefacts have
been found to the left of the bridleway along here.
  Keep straight ahead and follow the bridleway for just over a mile into
Houghton Forest and along what is known as the Denture. A bridleway
leads off to the left but ignore this and keep straight ahead until you reach
a signed bridleway on the right.

5 Follow this grassy path to a field and then continue along the right-hand bridleway. There are more lovely views from here. As the woods open out keep walking along the bridleway as it takes you through a large field and then heads back into more woodland. When you reach a crossroads go left and follow the track downhill and back to the start point of the route.

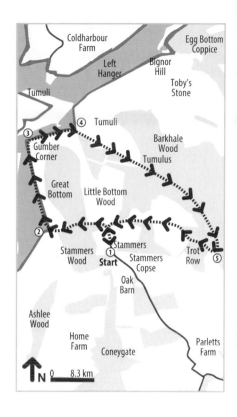

Points of interest

The faint banks and ditches of a Neolithic enclosure can be seen between points 3 and 4 (a couple of ridges in the landscape). The camp is one of five causewayed enclosures that can be found along the South Downs demonstrating Neolithic activity, with pottery and flint tools of the period (c.3000–2400 BCE) having been discovered here.

During the spring there are patches of bluebells scattered along the route.

Nuthurst

START St Andrew's church,
RH13 6LH, TQ192261

DISTANCE 3½ miles (5.6km)

SUMMARY An easy route on
footpaths and bridleways though
woodland and farmland

PARKING Roadside parking by
the church. Postcode: RH13 6LH

MAPS OS Explorer OL34;
Landranger 198

WHERE TO EAT AND DRINK The
Black Horse Inn is close to the
start and end point of the route
(www.theblackhorseinn.com)

A gentle walk through serene pine woodland and farmland surrounding the
village of Nuthurst.

1   From the church take the bridleway opposite. At the three-way
fingerpost continue along the tarmac bridleway as it swings round to the
left and then winds its way past some farm buildings.

2   As the tarmac path peters out at a junction, remain on the bridleway
leading into woodland. Keep to the main path as it leads you through
around a mile of magnificent pine woodland and eventually arrives at a
quiet lane.

3   At the lane turn left and then almost immediately take the bridleway
on the opposite side signed for Newells Rough. Follow the bridleway
through the woodland for approximately ½ mile before the path crosses a
stream and then leads back uphill. Keep straight ahead on the main path
along this stretch ignoring a sharp turn off to the left and another path to
the right leading into the woods. At a T-junction by a three-way sign, go
right.

4   At the next three-way fingerpost go right, dropping off the bridleway
and onto a public footpath. This leads down to a wooden footbridge and
back up to a gate leading into a field. Follow the footpath along the right-
hand edge of the field to another gate and then continue straight ahead,
walking steadily uphill until you reach a lane.

5 Turn right and very shortly after turn right again onto Prings Lane. After approximately 20yds go left over a stile. Follow this footpath through the next couple of fields and over the next stile. Bear right across a small field with a pond and climb another stile into a larger field. Go right and head diagonally across to another stile in the far corner.

6 Cross the stile and head back into woodland. At the T-junction go right and at the end of the path go through a gate to your left and cross the centre of the field. Once across turn right, following the footpath along the bottom edge to a gate. Follow the path for a short distance and then turn left and head back to the church.

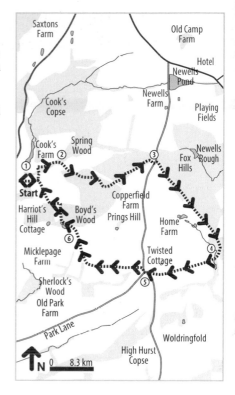

Points of interest

St Andrew's church at the start and end point of the walk is well worth a look. There is evidence of a church on this site since the twelfth century.

The woodlands around the village of Nuthurst are a great place to see bluebells during spring.

Harting Downs

START Harting Downs National Trust car park, GU31 5PN (nearest), SU791180

DISTANCE 3½ miles (5.7km) or 6½ miles (10.4km)

SUMMARY Two moderately challenging routes along bridleways, footpaths and byways involving some steep climbs

PARKING National Trust pay and display car park. Postcode: GU31 5PN

MAPS OS Explorer OL8; Landranger 197

WHERE TO EAT AND DRINK The Royal Oak pub is passed on the longer route (royaloakhooksway.co.uk/aboutus.html)

Two hilly routes within the South Downs National Park, offering fantastic panoramic views.

①   Leave the car park via the path opposite the information board and walk across a field towards a gate. At the gate take the bridleway straight ahead, then turn left heading downhill and turn right onto the South Downs Way. Remain straight ahead on the South Downs Way for almost a mile as it rises and falls.

②   At the bottom of a hill you reach a gate and crossroads. Follow the central path ahead, climbing steeply to the top of Beacon Hill, the site of an Iron Age hill fort. At the top go through the gate and continue straight ahead.

③a.   For the shorter route take a right-hand permissive path just after passing a trig point. Follow this down for around ½ mile then turn right onto the South Downs Way and rejoin the longer route at point 7.

③   Continue straight ahead past the trig point then bear slightly left. Follow the bridleway down through the stunning landscape. At the bottom of the hill the bridleway rejoins the South Downs Way and heads uphill to a gate by a cattle grid before descending again. At the bottom where the path forks, go left and then almost immediately turn right. Walk to a crossroads where you ignore restricted byway turnings and continue ahead taking the slightly raised path along the bottom edge of a field. Continue ahead for just under ½ mile, ignoring a left bridleway turning about halfway along.

4 At the T-junction, turn right onto the restricted byway. Once past the farm continue straight ahead for nearly ½ mile.

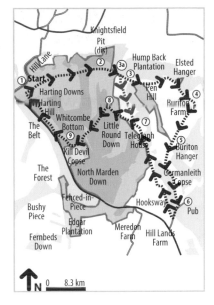

5 Just after a patch of woodland take a bridleway left through a gate running through the centre of a field to reach another gate. Walk through a meadow and then a wooded valley, continuing straight on to reach a road.

6 Turn right past the Royal Oak pub and head uphill. Take a restricted byway on the right and follow it for almost ½ mile, ignoring a footpath on the left when the byway bends. When the path forks by a gate, go left and walk past a house. This bridleway soon takes you along a tree-lined drive. Follow the drive past buildings and when it splits, bear right. At the next fork go right again, leaving the drive and following the bridleway ahead.

7 Go through a gate and when the path splits, take the South Downs Way left. Continue on this path for around ⅓ mile to a left bridleway.

8 Follow the left bridleway downhill to reach a crossroads by a dew pond. Take the footpath straight ahead, leading uphill into woodland.

9 At the next fingerpost turn right then soon after bear left with woods on your left and a meadow on the right. Follow the path along the edge of the meadow then continue straight ahead, ignoring a left footpath. Near the top, take a left footpath through a gate. Walk a short distance to meet another path then turn right and follow it back to the car park.

Points of interest

At the end of the walk you can see the eighteenth-century Vandalian Tower ahead of you. The folly is situated at the highest point of nearby National Trust property, Uppark.

START Saint Peter's church, Slinfold, RH13 0RR, TQ117315

DISTANCE 3½ miles (5.6km)

SUMMARY An easy route along quiet lanes, bridleways and footpaths

PARKING Roadside parking. Postcode: RH13 0RR

MAPS OS Explorer OL34; Landranger 198

WHERE TO EAT AND DRINK The Red Lyon Pub in the village is close to the start point of the walk (revivedinns.co.uk/redlyonslinfold)

A relaxing circular walk around the quiet lanes, woodland and farmland surrounding the pretty village of Slinfold, near Horsham.

① Take the public footpath to the right of the church and walk straight through the graveyard and then through an alleyway leading to a lane. Turn right at the lane and continue straight along the bridleway, ignoring a footpath off to the left, as it leads gently uphill to a large house on a corner.

② When you reach the gates of a house, turn right onto a woodland track and follow the bridleway downhill and then onto a narrow track running alongside a stream. Continue straight ahead along the main path, ignoring a turning off to the right. A footbridge soon takes you over the stream. Once over the bridge turn right and follow the bridleway along the bottom edge of a field. Keep straight ahead, ignoring any turnings, and when you reach Nowhurst Farm go straight ahead, walking along the lane.

③ After approximately ½ mile turn right onto a bridleway leading through woodland. Ignore any footpaths off to the left or right as you walk along here. The bridleway takes you through woods, across fields and then to another small footbridge. Once over the bridge, the path forks.

④ Bear right at the fork, crossing the grass, and then turn right onto a farm track and follow the bridleway past the farm. Once past the farm, ignore a footpath to the left and at the next junction go right. This leads you through a field to the left of a house and then into a small patch of woodland. Cross two small footbridges and then follow the footpath round to the right. This path winds its way through trees and farmland before arriving at a lane. Go left here and shortly after, at some office buildings, turn right and follow the footpath back to Saint Peter's church.

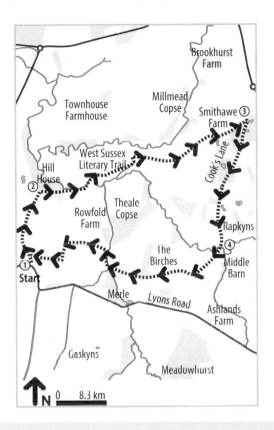

Points of Interest

 The picturesque village of Slinfold has a quintessentially English feel to it and is home to one of the oldest cricket clubs in Sussex, having been founded in 1775.

Part of this route follows a section of the West Sussex Literary Trail, a long distance trail (55 miles) running between Chichester in the south and Horsham in the north of the county. The route marks points along the way connected with famous literary figures such as Hilaire Belloc who had strong associations with West Sussex, and William Blake who lived for a time in Felpham and ended up in court in Chichester.

Ferring

START Amberley Drive (west of Aldsworth Avenue), Ferring, BN12 4QG, TQ106020

DISTANCE 3.5 miles (5.6km)

SUMMARY An easy walk following footpaths, bridleways, beachfront and roads

PARKING Free roadside parking on Amberley Drive. Postcode: BN12 4QG

MAPS OS Explorer OL10; Landranger 198

WHERE TO EAT AND DRINK The Bluebird Cafe (thebluebirdcafeferring.co.uk)

A gentle coastal route between Ferring and Goring-by-Sea.

(1) Start in Amberley Drive (west of Aldsworth Avenue) and locate the woodland path running alongside the Goring Gap. Follow the path north and when it forks by a playing field, go left. Cross the field diagonally heading to the far left corner and then follow the right edge of the next playing field to leave the recreation ground by the gate.

(2) Turn left and follow the tree-lined path (the Ilex Avenue) all the way to the end. Once at the end turn right onto Sea Lane and just after crossing Midhurst Drive, take a footpath leading past a cricket ground and Little Twitten Recreation Ground on the left side of the road. At the end of the path, turn right.

(3) Follow Ferring Street until you reach a library on the left-hand side. Take the alley just past the library then turn right and very soon left into Rife Way. Follow the residential road with a park to your right and then a recreation ground to your left. Continue to the end where you come to Ferring Country Centre. Turn left and follow the drive, ignoring a footpath turning at the first corner. Continue along the drive and at the entrance gates go left.

(4) Follow the footpath alongside the Ferring Rife. Keep straight ahead along this stretch, ignoring any footpath turnings (including a bridge over the rife) until you arrive at the Bluebird Cafe on the seafront.

(5) Turn left and follow the shingle path in front of the beach huts then continue along the tarmac path of Patterson's Walk with the beach to your

right (ignoring any footpath turnings off the main path). At the end of Patterson's Walk, continue straight ahead along the seafront footpath.

⑥ Just before you reach a toilet block on Goring Greensward, turn left and head away from the beach and through the trees. At the road cross over and continue ahead through the strip of woodland to arrive back at the start and end point of the walk.

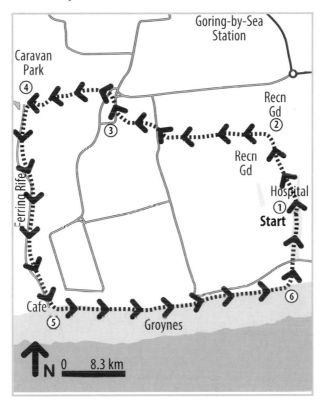

Points of interest

The Ilex Avenue is a tree-lined bridleway running between Goring and Ferring. The oak trees were planted in the nineteenth century by the inhabitants of Goring Hall to create carriage entrances to the estate. In 1935 the avenue was given to Worthing Borough Council in order to be used as 'a public walk and pleasure ground in perpetuity'.

Worth Way

START Burleigh Way car park, RH10 4UQ, TQ346373

DISTANCE 3¾ miles (6km)

SUMMARY An easy walk following footpaths and a stretch of the Worth Way; one short section of road

PARKING Free car park on Burleigh Way. Postcode: RH10 4UQ

MAPS OS Explorer OL135; Landranger 187

WHERE TO EAT AND DRINK The Carriage is close to the start and end point of the walk (thecarriage.org)

A circular walk following part of a disused railway line between Three Bridges and East Grinstead.

① From the Burleigh Way car park turn right. At the top of Burleigh Way, turn left and then go straight ahead following the private road (Sandhill Lane) signed for the Sussex Border Path. Follow the road past houses until you reach a footpath turning on the right.

② Remain on this footpath for almost ½ mile as it leads down to cross a stream and then heads back up again to eventually reach a T-junction by some buildings.

③ At the T-junction turn right. When you come to a drive, cross over and continue on for a short distance looking out for a footpath turning on the right. Take this footpath to a track. Then turn right (ignoring footpath sign straight ahead) and remain on the signed path for around ½ mile to reach a main road.

④ At the main road (North Street) turn right. Follow the road a short distance and then cross over (taking care) to take a footpath on the left. Follow the path to the right of a large house and then go through a gate and follow the access road for the reservoir. As the road bends left, follow the footpath straight ahead leading towards woodland.

⑤ Climb the stile and enter Hundred Acres wood. Continue along the signed footpath through the woodland, bearing right at the fork immediately after the stile, for nearly ½ mile, ignoring any tracks off the path as you go. When you emerge from the woods onto a drive, turn right.

This shortly takes you to Worth Way, a 7-mile accessible path between Three Bridges and East Grinstead running along an old disused railway line.

⑥ Turn right onto Worth Way, heading in the direction of East Grinstead. Follow the path along the old railway line for just over 1 mile back to Crawley Down. Worth Way emerges onto Old Station Road at Crawley Down. Follow the road past houses and shops back to the car park, the start and end point of the walk.

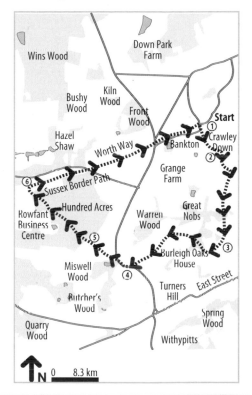

Points of interest

Worth Way is an accessible 7-mile-long path for walkers, horse-riders and cyclists opened in 1979. The path runs along an old railway line which used to connect Three Bridges and East Grinstead but was shut in the 1960s, a part of the Beeching rail closures. As it is mostly surfaced, it makes for an ideal route for wheelchair users and parents with buggies.

Slindon

START Nore Wood Lane, Slindon, BN18 0RJ, SU959098

DISTANCE 3¾ miles (5.9km) or 6 miles (9.7km)

SUMMARY Two moderate routes along woodland and farmland footpaths and bridleways

PARKING Lay-by parking at the start point. Postcode: BN18 0RJ

MAPS OS Explorer OL10; Landranger 197

WHERE TO EAT AND DRINK None en route; The Forge cafe and shop in Slindon village (www.slindonforge.com)

Two peaceful walks through the National Trust Slindon estate.

1 Facing the National Trust information sign, take the left bridleway. Walk through the woodland and past fields for approximately 1 mile, ignoring a turning to the left and continuing straight ahead at a crossroads. Continue past a metal gate and walk on to reach a junction with six paths going off it by a wooden bench.

2 From here take the bridleway signed to Upwaltham. Climb through woodland for just over ½ mile, ignoring any turnings off to the right. The bridleway is then joined by a forestry track. Continue uphill to a T-junction.

2 a. For the shorter route take the right bridleway signed to Bignor (Stane Street) and rejoin the longer route at point 6.

3 Turn right and follow the path ahead, ignoring a left bridleway. You soon emerge from woodland with the bridleway narrowing and leading through fields. Ignore a turning to the left and continue straight ahead admiring the views along this stretch.

4 Around 100yds past a bench carved from a large tree trunk, go left (uphill). Follow this bridleway up to where it crosses the South Downs Way and then continue straight ahead. The bridleway leads around the top of the hill and back down to reach the South Downs Way.

⑤ Go through a gate and then turn right onto the South Downs Way. After about 100yds, the bridleway is joined by another on the left and then immediately forks. Go left here, heading towards Gumber bothy. This path follows the remains of a Roman road, Stane Street, which once connected Chichester to London.

At a crossroads continue straight ahead and climb a stile, then continue along Stane Street for approximately ½ mile as it leads through fields, ignoring a left-hand turning by a stile. Continue downhill.

⑥ Follow the bridleway left (or right on the shorter route) towards Gumber Farm and bothy. Go through the farmyard and continue straight ahead through gates and back into the woods.

After approximately 250yds take a right-hand grassy footpath leading downhill. This path forks almost immediately. Go left and once at the bottom of the hill, turn left again. Follow the grassy path until you meet a junction with a bridleway.

⑦ Go left and walk uphill following the bridleway past fields and a National Trust wooden building. Head downhill and when you reach a crossroads turn right. Follow this bridleway, ignoring any paths off it, back to the start point.

Points of interest

The National Trust is running a long-term regeneration project in Northwood, Slindon. The scheme aims to return 185 acres of arable land to woodland and wooded pasture.

Kirdford

START St John the Baptist church, Glasshouse Lane, Kirdford, RH14 0LU, TQ018265

DISTANCE 3½ miles (5.5km)

SUMMARY A circular route along lanes, bridleways and footpaths

PARKING Roadside parking on Glasshouse Lane. Postcode: RH14 0LU

MAPS OS Explorer OL34; Landranger 197

WHERE TO EAT AND DRINK The Half Moon pub at the start and end of the walk (www.halfmoonkirdford.co.uk)

A circular walk in the countryside and woodland surrounding the pretty village of Kirdford. This walk is lined by bluebells in springtime.

① Begin with the Half Moon pub to your left and follow the road round to the right walking past a cricket pitch until you arrive at Boxall Stud.

② Turn left and walk through Boxall Stud's yard and then along an avenue of trees with paddocks either side. At the fork go right and follow the path to woodland. Continue straight ahead until you reach a drive with a large industrial unit to your left. Cross over and take the bridleway opposite.

③ Head down through the woodland to cross Boxal Brook, then turn left. When you arrive at a metal gate, swing left and follow the broad path leading through Barkfold Rough. The bridleway begins to climb to reach a house by a crossroads.

④ Go left and take the footpath with a view of Blackdown Hill ahead of you. Bear right at the barn and follow the well-defined path between hedges as it zigzags its way through farmland before arriving at a field.

⑤ Cross the field to a drive. Turn left onto the drive for a few paces before almost immediately turning right. Follow the footpath along the right-hand side of a field. Turn left at the corner and follow the signed path through hedges and under wires.

At the next field turn right, then shortly after, at an oak tree, go left. There's a fence and hedge running to your right along this footpath. About halfway across there's a gap with another handmade footpath sign pointing into woodland. Go right here.

6 Go down steps, across a bridge and up the other side. Follow the path with the field to your right. When you arrive at another footbridge and gate go straight ahead through the gate, ignoring the right-hand turning.

7 Walk along the left side of the meadow, then dip into woodland and head to a gate. Go through and continue along the signed footpath winding through the woodland. Cross a footbridge, climb some steps and then continue past a field.

8 At a three-way fingerpost go left following the footpath to a drive, which leads you between fences back to the village. At the road turn left and return to the church.

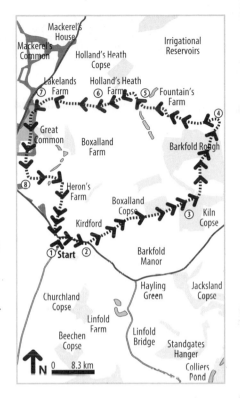

Littlehampton and Climping

START West Beach car park,
Rope Walk, Littlehampton,
BN17 5DL, TQ026017

DISTANCE 3¾ miles (6km)

SUMMARY A circular route through
farmland and along a stretch of beach

PARKING Pay and display car park at
the start point. Postcode: BN17 5DL

MAPS OS Explorer OL10;
Landranger 197

WHERE TO EAT AND DRINK
West Beach Cafe in the car park
at the start and end point

A coastal walk taking in a quiet, unspoilt stretch of beach between Climping and
Littlehampton.

1   Take the public footpath leading out of the West Beach car park
walking away from the sea and follow the path with Littlehampton
Harbour to your right and a golf course to your left. This area feels quite
industrial but the views over the River Arun make it an interesting stroll.

2   When you reach a footpath leading down an alleyway, turn left and
follow it to a raised bank skirting the edge of a golf course. This footpath
winds through trees and tall reeds for approximately ¾ mile. Be warned,
this stretch can become overgrown and difficult to traverse, especially in
late summer.

3   At a three-way fingerpost turn right, walking away from the golf
course and follow the footpath for approximately ½ mile until you arrive
at a field. Continue straight across the field to a crossroads by a small
bridge crossing a rife and then continue straight ahead into the next field.
As you near a thatched cottage, the footpath bears left and leads to a wide
grassy path. Go right here and walk a short distance until you reach the
flint wall of an old barn, now converted into a house (Lower Dairy Barn).

4   At the barn turn left and cross the field, then at the wide track go left
again and follow the byway running between fields all the way down to
the beach.

⑤ Once you arrive at the beach, turn left and follow the shoreline eastwards back to West Beach car park. This stretch first takes you along Climping beach, with its decaying timber groynes and the remnants of an old sea wall which have all been battered by storms in recent years, and then leads you on to West Beach, a Local Nature Reserve and one of only two sand dune systems in West Sussex. As you near the end of the route, the remains of a Napoleonic fort can be seen to your left.

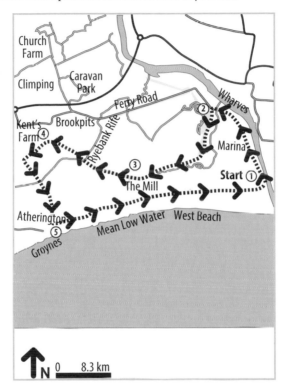

Points of interest

West Beach and Climping beach are nationally protected Sites of Special Scientific Interest (SSSI) due to the sand dunes, sand flats and vegetated shingle on the foreshore and a small patch of salt marsh found along the coast there. It's also one of the only stretches of shoreline in the county backed by fields rather than buildings and roads and makes for an ever-changing dramatic landscape due to coastal erosion.

Horsted Keynes

START Recreation ground car park, RH17 7AF, TQ383281

DISTANCE 3¾ miles (6km)

SUMMARY A moderate undulating walk mainly along footpaths, with some bridleways and lanes and a short section of busy road

PARKING Recreation ground car park at the start. Postcode: RH17 7AF

MAPS OS Explorer 135; Landranger 187

WHERE TO EAT AND DRINK The Green Man pub, close to the start and end point (greenmanhorstedkeynes.co.uk)

A circular walk around Horsted Keynes with views of steam trains chugging up and down the Bluebell Railway line.

1 From the car park, head to the main road and take the footpath opposite walking towards the church. Follow the path downhill, which joins Church Lane. Once past the church and school, take a left footpath leading downhill through woodland. This winds around an old house before arriving by a lake. Go straight ahead at the crossroads and walk through the trees to reach a lane.

2 Turn right onto the lane, walk a short distance and then take the footpath over a stile on the left. Follow the footpath diagonally uphill across the field to the top right corner, then climb another stile, go right and through a farm.

Once in the farmyard, look out for a farmer's sign pointing to Nobles Farm and follow this through a gate into a field, with a short walk to another gate leading onto a track. Go straight ahead for around 200yds to a bridge crossing the Bluebell Railway line.

3 Once across, continue straight ahead with trees to your right. After approximately 250yds there is a footpath turning in the corner of the field. Turn left in front of the stile and head up, keeping the hedge and farmhouse to your right, then continue downhill, crossing a stile on the right. The path leads you alongside the railway line and then to a road.

4 Turn left at the road under the railway bridge and walk for around 60yds, taking care as it can be busy. Take a right footpath heading through

trees and then across a field to join a track at the top. Follow this track for about ½ mile until you climb up towards a building where the path turns sharp right. At this corner take the kissing gate to the left, crossing a field to join Treemans Road.

⑤ At the road turn left. Walk around 50yds then turn right onto another footpath. Walk downhill to woodland. Cross a stile and a stream and then head back uphill to a T-junction with a bridleway. Turn left.

⑥ Follow the bridleway back to Horsted Keynes. When the path forks bear left, remaining on the Sussex Border Path. The bridleway leads to a lane that twists round to the left and leads to a crossroads with another lane. Go straight ahead here and follow Chapel Lane back to the start point.

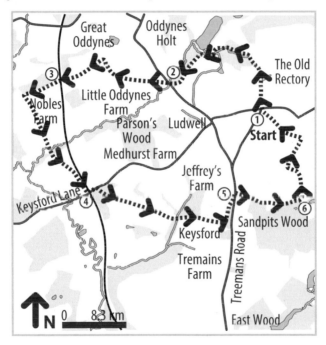

Points of interest

The Bluebell Railway, which has a station at Horsted Keynes, is a preserved heritage steam train line that runs between Sheffield Park and East Grinstead.

Chanctonbury Ring

START Chanctonbury Ring Road car park, BN44 3DN, TQ145124

DISTANCE 3¾ miles (6.1km)

SUMMARY A moderate walk along footpaths and bridleways through woodland with a fairly steep climb up to an Iron Age hill fort

PARKING Free car park (small). Postcode: BN44 3DN

MAPS OS Explorer OL10; Landranger 198

WHERE TO EAT AND DRINK None en route

The steep climb up to this (supposedly haunted) Iron Age hill fort is well worth it for the panoramic views you get from the top.

① From the car park, walk straight ahead uphill ignoring turnings off either side. Go past a metal gate and a reservoir to your right and head fairly steeply up the stony track through woodland. Follow the path as it curves round to the left onto a bridleway and continue uphill through Chalkpit Wood.

② At the top of the hill you arrive at a crossroads where the South Downs Way meets the bridleway. Turn right onto the South Downs Way and head towards Chanctonbury Ring, distinctive by the clump of beech trees on top of the Iron Age hill fort. Follow the path around the lower edge of Chanctonbury Ring. From up here you get stunning panoramic views across the Downs and over to the Isle of Wight. Continue along the south side of the Ring and walk towards a gate.

③ Once past the gate, leave the South Downs Way and take the bridleway passing Chanctonbury dew pond on your right. Walk across a field that begins to lead downhill and then go through the gate on the opposite side. Follow the chalk path steeply downhill. The track narrows and follows the line of a wire fence to your right before arriving at another gate, which briefly takes you back out onto the South Downs Way. Walk for a short distance, then take a right turning onto a bridleway which enters a field through a gate.

④ Cross the field, then pass through another gate and head into the woodland. Keep straight ahead, sticking to this bridleway through the woods and ignoring any turnings off to the left or right.

⑤ At a fork bear right through the metal gate, keeping the field and wire fence to your left. The path leads you back to Chanctonbury Ring Road, where you turn left to head back to the car park.

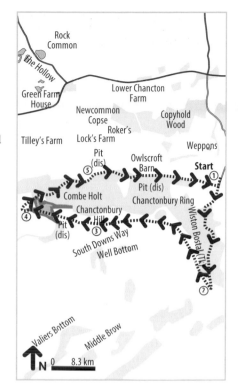

Points of interest

Chanctonbury Ring is an Iron Age hill fort and has a rich and interesting history. During Elizabethan times a beacon was erected on the top of the Ring to warn of the Spanish Armada. The beech trees growing at the top were first planted in 1760 by then landowner, Charles Goring. Most of them were blown down during the 1987 hurricane but have since been replanted.

The Ring is also said to be haunted. The writer Robert Macfarlane spent the night up there and wrote that he was awoken by what sounded like human screams in the middle of the night.

Chattri Memorial

START Braypool Lane parking bays, Patcham, BN1 8YF, TQ302094

DISTANCE 4 miles (6.2km)

SUMMARY A moderate walk following bridleways and lanes

PARKING Free roadside parking by start point. Postcode: BN1 8YF

MAPS OS Explorer OL11; Landranger 198

WHERE TO EAT AND DRINK None en route

A walk on the West Sussex border taking in far-reaching views and an Indian war memorial on the downs.

1   From the parking bays on Braypool Lane take the bridleway (Sussex Border Path) through the gate signed to Chattri. Follow the grassy path up through the centre of the field. The views quickly begin to open out all around and the white marble memorial can soon be seen ahead of you. Continue on through the next field (there are sometimes cattle grazing here) and then, as you near the monument, another path veers off to the right. Take this path and go through the gate to visit Chattri.

2   Once you've visited the memorial, walk back to the bridleway and turn right through a gate to continue on in the direction you were headed. After just over ½ mile you will reach a crossroads.

3   When you arrive at a gate by the crossroads, leave the Sussex Border Path and turn right. Follow this bridleway as it weaves its way down and takes you through a gate. The path continues past a brick barn and on a short distance to reach another crossroads by a large farm building.

4   At the crossroads take the bridleway right, following the path steeply uphill and then along the edge of a field. As the path nears a farmhouse it swings left and reaches a farm track. Bear right here and then follow the bridleway for just under ½ mile through fields, heading down to reach a gate into access land. Go through the gate and continue downhill walking past a rifle range and out to a lane.

⑤ Bear right onto the quiet lane and follow it all the way back down to Braypool Lane, enjoying views over Brighton as you go. After just under ½ mile you will arrive back at the start point of the walk.

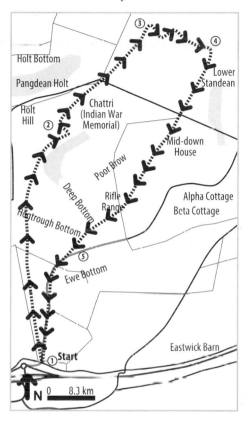

Points of interest

Chattri is a memorial to commemorate the thousands of Indian soldiers who lost their lives serving alongside British forces during the First World War. Fifty-three Hindu and Sikh men died in Brighton hospitals during the conflict and were taken up to the South Downs to be cremated in line with their tradition.

The marble monument was built in 1920 and stands on the spot on the South Downs where the men were cremated. All those who served are still remembered in a memorial service at Chattri each year.

START St John the Divine church,
Patching, BN13 3XF, TQ087064

DISTANCE 4 miles (6.2km)

SUMMARY A circular route
along woodland and farmland
footpaths, bridleways and lanes

PARKING Roadside parking at the
start point. Postcode: BN13 3XF

MAPS OS Explorer OL10;
Landranger 197

WHERE TO EAT AND DRINK
None en route; the World's End
pub is close to the start point
(worldsendpatching.co.uk)

A circular woodland walk with bluebells in springtime and wide-reaching views
from Patching Hill.

[1] From the church, follow the concrete track past a gate and farm
buildings to a field. Take the footpath straight ahead, walking towards a
wood. Climb a stile and follow the footpath straight ahead through the
trees and then across a field. At the crossroads keep straight ahead until
you reach a farm track leading to a lane.

[2] Turn left at the lane and walk past a farm, then take the footpath on
the right. Follow the path for around ¼ mile as it leads across fields and
behind a cottage, until you reach a junction with a bridleway.

[3] Turn right onto the bridleway and follow it along the lane leading
gently uphill until you arrive at a T-junction with another bridleway.

[4] Go right here and follow the bridleway as it continues uphill and
leads into woodland. When you arrive at a crossroads soon after, continue
straight ahead and then continue on through the woods for around
⅓ mile. Towards the end of this stretch you will come to a four-way
junction. Continue ahead on the bridleway for a short distance to where
the path splits three ways.

[5] At the junction go right and follow the bridleway through the trees.
Continue for nearly ½ mile, ignoring any forestry track turnings and a
footpath on the left as you go.

[6] When you get to a bridleway crossroads turn right, then at the next crossroads soon after continue straight ahead. Go through a gate leaving Angmering Park Estate. The trees begin to thin out and the landscape opens up. The broad grassy path soon forks but it doesn't matter which side you take, as they meet up again a bit further along. There are great views along this stretch.

[7] When you reach a junction by a gate take the bridleway right and walk along the top edge of the field. About halfway along, turn left to follow the footpath going directly across towards the church spire.

Once at the bottom, turn left and head back to the start point.

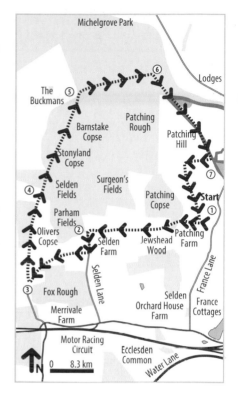

Points of interest

The church of St John the Divine, which marks the beginning and end point of the walk, is a thirteenth-century church that was restored in 1889 and is well worth a visit.

Beeding Hill

START Beeding Hill National Trust car park, Mill Hill, BN43 5FB (near), TQ207096

DISTANCE 4 miles (6.2km)

SUMMARY A moderate hilly walk following footpaths and bridleways

PARKING Free car park at the start. Postcode: BN43 5FB (near)

MAPS OS Explorer OL11; Landranger 198

WHERE TO EAT AND DRINK Cafe at Truleigh Hill Youth Hostel (www.yha.org.uk/hostel/yha-truleigh-hill)

A walk up on the South Downs north of Shoreham, with fantastic views out to sea.

① Take the bridleway heading out of the back of the car park past the silver National Trust Beeding Hill car park sign. Follow the narrow path downhill between steep banks either side. Ignore a gate into an access lane on the left and a right-hand footpath up some steps and continue along the bridleway as it narrows and heads under trees. The path eventually curves around to the left with open fields and great countryside views opening up. Continue walking to reach a footpath turning on the right, leading uphill alongside a fence.

② Follow this path up to a gate leading into a field and continue climbing steeply. At the top of the hill you come to a T-junction. Go left and follow the bridleway along the edge of the hill to reach another gate. Go through this and continue ahead bearing slight right following the bridleway uphill. There are more fantastic views to enjoy along this stretch.

③ The path soon leads to a right-hand bridleway turning. Take this and head up, bearing right as you climb to reach a lane and the South Downs Way.

④ When you reach the lane, turn left and follow the South Downs Way towards the youth hostel (where there is a cafe, toilets and water re-fill station). Once past the youth hostel continue in the same direction following the South Downs Way uphill. Just after a turning on the right for a house you will arrive at a crossroads where you turn right.

⑤ Follow the bridleway past barns and buildings to a gate. Go through and continue along the fenced-in path with fields either side for 1 mile, enjoying the sea views ahead as you go.

⑥ When you reach a junction by a set of gates turn right and follow the bridleway (the Monarch's Way) downhill between fences. Remain on this path for just over a mile. It leads downhill, then climbs back up and finally descends again before arriving back at the car park and the start point of the walk.

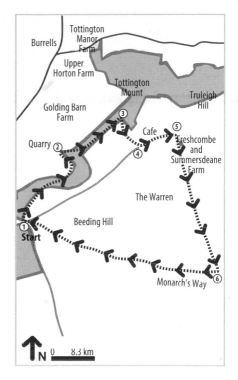

Points of interest

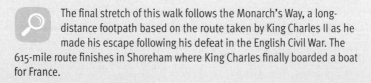

The final stretch of this walk follows the Monarch's Way, a long-distance footpath based on the route taken by King Charles II as he made his escape following his defeat in the English Civil War. The 615-mile route finishes in Shoreham where King Charles finally boarded a boat for France.

Shermanbury

START Quiet car park, Shermanbury, BN5 9AL, TQ211180

DISTANCE 4 miles (6.2km)

SUMMARY An easy walk following footpaths, bridleways and lanes; can be muddy and wet after rain

PARKING Free car park at the start point. Postcode: BN5 9AL

MAPS OS Explorer OL11; Landranger 198

WHERE TO EAT AND DRINK The Bull Inn is close to the start point (thebullinnhenfield.co.uk)

A lovely walk through the meadows and farmland surrounding the River Adur in Shermanbury.

1 Leave the car park and follow the grass verge to the Bull Inn. Cross the road and take the footpath opposite leading down steps, through a gate and over a footbridge. Cross the field bearing left and on the opposite side take the signed path right into the next field. Follow the left edge of this field to a gate, then continue straight ahead across another field to reach a junction of footpaths.

2 At the junction go straight ahead through the gate and over a footbridge. Follow the footpath straight ahead through the meadows for ⅓ mile. The path leads to a gate into a field. Cross the field, then at the T-junction go left and follow the top edge of the field to another gate. Go through this and over a footbridge, then continue straight ahead following the path between hedgerows and soon through a kissing gate. The path then leads along the edge of woodland and to the river.

3 At the river turn right and climb a stile into a field. Remain on this footpath as it follows the course of the Adur for around ¾ mile. When you reach a metal gate bear left to cross the stile and continue on to reach a bridge.

4 Cross the footbridge and go through the gate to access the bridge over the river. Turn left on the other side, following the riverbank in the opposite direction. Take the next footpath on the right over the bridge. Cross the field bearing right to reach a road.

⑤ Turn left and follow the lane past the church and round to the right. When the road bends right again, take the bridleway on the left along a private road. After just under ¼ mile the bridleway forks off to the left and continues along a track.

⑥ After ½ mile the bridleway veers right passing a house and some farm buildings. Continue along the bridleway past St Giles church, Shermanbury and when you reach a crossroads keep straight ahead. This leads you to metal gates leading out to the main road.

⑦ Go left and follow the footpath alongside the road over the bridge and back towards the pub and car park.

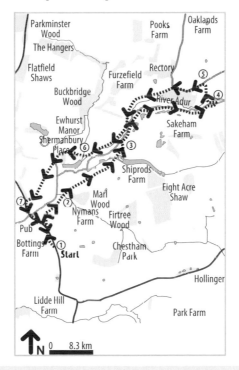

Points of interest

Shermanbury cemetery was created in 1888 as an extra burial ground for nearby twelfth-century St Giles church. The tiny chapel was built in order to conduct pauper funerals.

Wisborough Green

START St Peter Ad Vincula
church, RH14 0EA, TQ051258

DISTANCE 4 miles (6.2km)

SUMMARY An easy route along
footpaths and bridleways with a
short stretch along a main road

PARKING Roadside parking close to
the start point. Postcode: RH14 0EA

MAPS OS Explorer OL34;
Landranger 197

WHERE TO EAT AND DRINK The
Three Crowns pub is very close
to the start and end point of the
route (thethreecrownsinn.com)

A varied walk through Wisborough Green, taking in a stretch of the canal and the
River Arun.

1 From the church, take the public footpath heading past the
churchyard and towards the main road. Cross over and follow the
bridleway along Harsfold Lane, walking past some allotments and keeping
straight ahead. When you reach a fork with another bridleway, bear left.
Go through two gates and cross the River Arun, then continue on until
you reach a crossroads.

2 Once at the crossroads climb the stile on the left-hand side and
follow the path running along the edge of the canal (the Old Wey and
Arun Canal). Continue on this path until you reach a bridge where you
cross the water and then continue walking in the same direction on the
opposite side of the canal.

3 Ignore any footpaths off to the right, keeping to the waterside path
which leads you over the river via two footbridges. Go through a gate
and along the edge of a meadow before crossing another footbridge and
arriving at Lording's Lock and a waterwheel. Once past the lock climb
a stile and follow the path straight ahead through a meadow to reach
another stile.

4 Follow the footpath to the left keeping the river to your right. Go
through a patch of woodland then cross another meadow to reach a
bridge and a crossroads.

5 Go left at the crossroads, then cross the field to reach the main road. Climb the stile and turn left at the A-road then follow the verge for around 100yds (the road can be busy so take care along this short stretch). Cross over and climb a stile to take a permissive footpath on the opposite side. Follow it left.

6 The permissive path soon joins a public footpath. Follow the signed footpath as it winds its way through fields and farmland heading back to the St Peter Ad Vincula church. When you get to a crossroads, keep straight ahead along the footpath. You soon get to a stile leading back into the churchyard, the start and end point of the route.

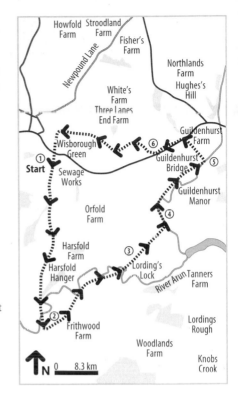

Henfield

START Hollands Lane,
BN5 9UL, TQ206159

DISTANCE 4 miles (6.5km)

SUMMARY A circular route on
bridleways and riverside footpaths

PARKING Roadside parking on
Hollands Lane. Postcode: BN5 9UL

MAPS OS Explorer OL11;
Landranger 198

WHERE TO EAT AND DRINK None
en route; a selection of places
to eat and drink in Henfield

A relaxing circular route from Henfield and along the banks of the River Adur.

1 Starting from the top of Hollands Lane (close to the junction with Lower Station Road), locate the signed Downs Link path and head up the track.

As part of the Downs Link path, this first section of the walk follows the route of an old disused railway line closed in the 1960s. There is evidence of its prior use along the way, such as the remnants of an old railway bridge. Keep straight ahead for just over 1½ miles, ignoring any turnings off to the left or right, until you reach a bridge crossing the River Adur.

2 When you reach the river, cross the bridge and take the right-hand bridleway, which follows the route of the Adur as it meanders through farmland. Be aware there are sometimes cows grazing along this stretch depending on the time of year. Keep to this footpath remaining straight ahead and ignoring a bridleway on the left leading away from the river after approximately ½ mile of walking. Continue along the riverbank footpath for around a further ¾ mile until you arrive at another bridge (Bineham Bridge) crossing the water.

3 At the bridge turn right onto a bridleway, and once over the Adur, follow the path as it swings round to the left. At a gate follow the bridleway to the right as it leads away from the river and through the farmyard of New Inn Farm. Once through the farm continue to follow a surfaced lane leading gently uphill to reach a crossroads.

4 At the crossroads continue straight ahead remaining on the bridleway and ignoring any left or right turnings as you go for almost a mile. You will walk past an old cottage on the left and then cross a farm drive at Buckwish Farm before arriving back at Hollands Lane, the start and end point of the walk.

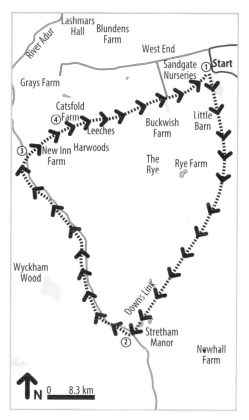

Points of interest

The Downs Link is a 37-mile long route linking Surrey and the North Downs to Shoreham-by-Sea and the South Downs. It follows the route of an old railway line that was closed in the 1960s and is today used by cyclists, walkers and horse riders.

New Inn Farm is named as such because there used to be a riverside pub on the site which served fishermen and river tradesmen between 1729 and 1916.

Blackdown

START National Trust car park, Tennyson's Lane, GU27 3BJ, SU920308

DISTANCE 4 miles (6.5km)

SUMMARY A moderate walk mainly on woodland and heathland footpaths and bridleways

PARKING National Trust car park. Postcode: GU27 3BJ

MAPS OS Explorer OL33; Landranger 186

WHERE TO EAT AND DRINK None en route

A fantastic walk across heathland and through woods with the best views across West Sussex.

1 Leave the car park via the roadside entrance and turn immediately left, following the bridleway to a gate and then to a junction with a wide clear path. Turn left. Follow the sunken path to a fork, then go right to follow the Sussex Border Path. At the next fingerpost turn right.

2 Follow the broad path to another fork, then bear left continuing along the Sussex Border Path. Continue straight ahead, ignoring a left turn, to reach a crossroads where you keep straight ahead through the gate. Shortly after, the path forks – go left and head downhill.

3 At the T-junction leave the Sussex Border Path and head left through a gate. Follow the bridleway downhill with steep banks either side. The bridleway swings right and leads past a house. Cross the drive and take the bridleway opposite.

4 At the lane turn left, then shortly after turn right and follow the byway along a lane signed for Sheetlands. Ignore a left turn into private woodland and continue over the hill. Take the left bridleway leading into woodland which soon swings right following a grassy path alongside a house before heading back into woodland. Ignore a right-hand footpath just past the house and continue ahead. When the path forks, go left and follow the bridleway leading gently uphill.

5 At the T-junction go left and follow the bridleway uphill. At the top keep straight ahead and then descend to a road. Turn left. Walk past stables, then take the bridleway on the right.

6 Follow the lane to a set of gates on the right with a bridleway leading back into Blackdown. The broad grassy path leads steadily uphill and soon becomes sandy underfoot as woodland gives way to heath. When the path meets the Serpent Trail, continue straight ahead. At the next junction walk straight ahead to the Temple of the Winds viewing point.

7 After taking in the stunning views, retrace your steps back to the broad bridleway, then go right. Walk through the trees and ignore a path on the left, then at the three-way fingerpost keep straight ahead. Shortly after when the path forks, go right. At a junction just before a National Trust notice board, turn right and follow the path back to the car park.

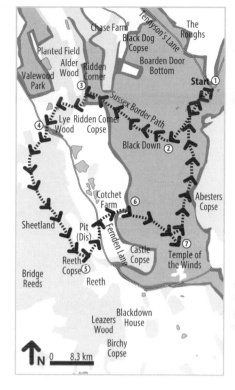

Temple of the Winds is named after a Bronze Age circular bank and offers one of the best views in the whole of West Sussex.

Heyshott and Cocking

START St James church, Heyshott,
GU29 0DJ, SU896181

DISTANCE 4 miles (6.5km)

SUMMARY A moderate walk along
footpaths and bridleways through
woodland, farmland and villages;
one very steep climb and descent

PARKING Free roadside
parking. Postcode: GU29 0DJ

MAPS OS Explorer OL8;
Landranger 197

WHERE TO EAT AND DRINK The
Unicorn Inn is close to the start
(unicorn-inn-heyshott.co.uk)

The steep climb is well worth it for the views and atmosphere from the top of
Heyshott Down.

1. Starting with St James church to your left, take the quiet lane forking
off to the right in front of you. Just past Cobden Club village hall turn
left onto the footpath signed for the New Lipchis Way, a 39-mile trail
running between Liphook and Chichester Harbour. Follow the path as it
runs along the edge of a field, then over a footbridge and across another
couple of fields, before leading up a small bank between hedges. Turn left
and then almost immediately right and follow the path uphill towards
Heyshott Down. At a gate turn right and continue uphill. This section
soon becomes very steep so take care along here. At the top of the hill
cross a gated field and turn right onto the South Downs Way.

2. After approximately 20yds go through a gate on the right and follow
the path diagonally through a field. The views along this stretch are
spectacular and make the climb well worth it. At the opposite end of the
field go through the gate and turn right heading downhill towards woods.
Skirt the bottom edge of the field and then go right, through a gate. The
path leads very steeply downhill through the woodland and continues
along the edge of a field. Approximately halfway across the field, before
you reach the farmhouse, turn left (keep your eyes peeled as it's easy to
miss this turning). Cross the field then descend some steps and turn left
onto a quiet lane.

③ Follow the lane and then walk directly through the churchyard and out to the lane beyond where you continue straight ahead past some buildings. At the adjoining road turn right following the footpath down a gravel drive, past some houses and then along an alley. The footpath runs alongside a bank and then turns right up some steps, taking you back out to farmland. Cross two fields, then follow the signed footpath leading diagonally across the third field towards a copse.

④ Walk through the patch of woodland and then continue on the same footpath as it leads through more farmland and over a couple of footbridges until you reach a lane. Go left here, following the lane back to the church.

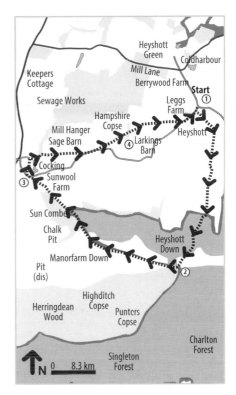

Points of interest

St Catherine of Siena church in Cocking is found midway through the route. Parts of the church date back to the eleventh century, however it's thought there was originally a wooden church on the site dating back to 680.

START The Bolney Stage, London Road, Bolney, RH17 5RL, TQ265238

DISTANCE 4 miles (6.5km)

SUMMARY A hilly circular route along lanes, bridleways and footpaths through woodland and farmland. Can be muddy in places

PARKING Roadside parking on London Road. Postcode: RH17 5RL

MAPS OS Explorer OL34; Landranger 198

WHERE TO EAT AND DRINK The Bolney Stage pub at the start and end of the walk (brunningandprice. co.uk/bolneystage/)

A varied hilly walk through woodland and farmland, offering fantastic views.

① With your back to the Bolney Stage, cross the road and take the footpath opposite walking straight ahead alongside a wire fence. When you reach a junction go right and follow the footpath through the woodland (can be muddy after wet weather). Cross a footbridge.

Just after another small bridge over a stream, you emerge from the woods. Continue along the footpath leading gradually uphill. When you reach a small lane, cross over and enter a field opposite following the footpath diagonally up towards the farmhouse.

② At the lane turn left. Ignore a footpath going off to the right and continue to a junction with another lane. Go right and follow this quiet road past Warninglid Water Tower.

③ Take the next footpath on the left through a gate and into a field. The path leads you downhill to a gate on the opposite side. Go through and follow the footpath past a pond to another field.

④ At a cottage by a road, turn immediately left taking a bridleway along a drive. Take the bridleway running to the left of the house which soon follows a lane uphill. Continue straight ahead to a farm, turn left and then right following the bridleway as it zigzags around the farm. Continue straight ahead for around ½ mile.

5 At the next farm continue straight ahead through a gate and then immediately turn right following the bridleway along the drive. When the drive meets a lane, go left. Ignore a footpath on the right and continue along the lane passing a junction with another lane on the left. Just past this, take a left footpath into woods.

6 Follow the footpath through the woods and then at the fork go right. This path skirts the grounds of a house and then takes you back into woodland. Follow this signed path back to the junction with the High Weald Landscape Trail path you encountered earlier. Here, turn left and then almost immediately right, following the footpath back to the Bolney Stage.

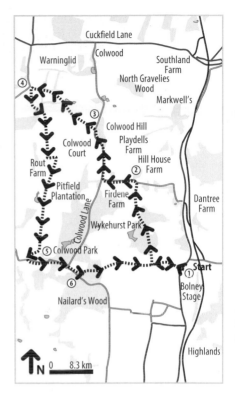

Points of interest

Part of this route goes through Wykehurst Park. Although not clearly seen on the route the estate is the grounds of a grand old 105-room Gothic Revival mansion that has appeared in many films over the years such as *The Eagle Has Landed* as well as three Hammer Horror films.

START Bramber public car park, BN44 3WE, TQ188106

DISTANCE 4 miles (6.6km)

SUMMARY A figure-of-eight walk along footpaths and quiet lanes. Riverside walking, so can get muddy

PARKING Free public car park with toilets (room for approximately twenty cars). Postcode: BN44 3WE

MAPS OS Explorer OL11; Landranger 198

WHERE TO EAT AND DRINK The Castle Inn Hotel is at the start and end point (castleinnhotel.co.uk)

Explore the remains of a castle and visit the oldest Norman church in Sussex on this riverside walk in Bramber.

1 At the car park entrance turn right and walk along the road heading towards the castle ruins. You will soon see some steps on your right. Climb these to see the remains of the Norman castle and to visit St Nicholas church, the oldest Norman church in Sussex. After you have explored the English Heritage site retrace your steps back down to the road and turn right. At the roundabout turn right again onto Castle Lane and follow it to the end, where you turn right onto a signed footpath.

2 Follow this footpath past the back of some houses to a gate. Once through the gate, continue along the footpath along the banks of a stream to a metal kissing gate. Turn right here, crossing the stream and walk towards a bridge over the River Adur.

3 Once over the bridge take the footpath straight ahead leading through a field. This will eventually lead you past a pond and some paddocks before a slightly rickety footbridge leads you to a gate and through a small field used for livestock. On the opposite side of the field go through a metal kissing gate and turn left at the T-junction.

4 Pass the farm to your left, cross a stile and then follow the footpath alongside a stream to your left for approximately ¾ mile, crossing multiple stiles and footbridges as you go.

5 At the river, turn left and continue along the footpath on the raised bank as it meanders back to the bridge crossing the Adur (point 3). Once back at the bridge continue straight ahead along the riverbank. Shortly after the bridge, the path forks. If you wish to make a short detour here to visit St Peter's church, take the left fork leading uphill. Otherwise, keep straight ahead.

6 Continue along the riverbank until you reach a road bridge. Turn right and walk back through the village to the start point. You will pass St Mary's House and gardens on your left along here, a medieval pilgrims' inn built around 1450.

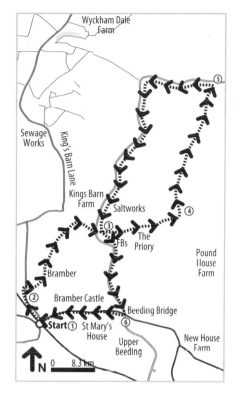

Points of interest

Bramber Castle is a Norman motte and bailey castle, built around 1073 and held by the de Braose family until 1450. It was briefly confiscated by King John in the early thirteenth century who accused owner, William de Braose, of disloyalty. Along with the castle, King John captured his wife and two sons who then died of starvation while being held at Windsor Castle.

Warnham

START St Margaret's church, Church Street, Warnham, RH12 3QW, TQ157336

DISTANCE 4 miles (6.5km)

SUMMARY An easy walk following footpaths, bridleways and lanes

PARKING Roadside parking near the church. Postcode: RH12 3QW

MAPS OS Explorer OL34; Landranger 187

WHERE TO EAT AND DRINK The Sussex Oak is close to the start and end point (www.thesussexoak.co.uk)

An interesting walk from the village of Warnham through surrounding countryside and a deer park.

① With your back to the church turn right, walk for a few paces and then take the signed public footpath opposite. The path leads to a primary school. At the school continue straight ahead on the footpath, passing the school to your right. This leads out to Lucas Road and a housing estate. Follow Lucas Road ahead ignoring Freeman Road on the right and Hollands Way on the left. When you reach Tillets Lane, cross over and take the footpath opposite. Follow the footpath straight on uphill, ignoring paths to the left and right, crossing two fields.

② In the far right-hand corner of the second field, go through a gap in the trees and head straight on with a line of trees to your right. The path leads to a crossroads with a bridleway. Turn left onto the bridleway and follow it downhill through woodland to Warnham Manor. The bridleway skirts the Manor and crosses a lake before reaching the main gates of the Manor.

③ Turn left and follow the lane for around 100yds, then take a footpath on the right heading diagonally uphill. Follow this footpath for around ¼ mile until you arrive at Byfleets Lane. Turn right and follow the lane to where a footpath crosses it.

④ Turn left onto the footpath and follow the trail down through several deer pens to a farm. At the next lane cross over and continue along the Sussex Literary Trail opposite as it takes you into Warnham Park. The path leads you through the deer park and on to Robin Hood Lane. Turn left at the lane.

⑤ Follow the lane for around ½ mile ignoring the footpath turnings off to the right where the road bends sharp left. As you near a busy roundabout, turn left onto a bridleway through gates and follow it along a tarmacked path. This leads to woods and a pond. Continue ahead through the trees to reach a footpath turning on the left just as the wall of the deer park grounds ends.

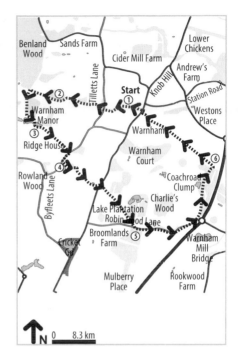

⑥ Take this footpath and follow it back towards Warnham. The path eventually opens into a field and then joins a wide track. Go left and follow this bridleway until it turns sharp right when you take the small footpath straight ahead. This path leads you back to the village, emerging just by the church.

Points of interest

The walk goes through a deer park attached to Warnham Court, which was a grand country home and estate built in 1826. As such there's a good chance of seeing plenty of deer along the way.

Standen House

START Hilltop Shaw car park by Standen House, West Hoathly Road, RH19 4NG, TQ385358

DISTANCE 4 miles (6.5km)

SUMMARY An easy walk following footpaths, bridleways and lanes

PARKING Hilltop Shaw public car park (free). Postcode: RH19 4NG

MAPS OS Explorer 135; Landranger 187

WHERE TO EAT AND DRINK The Old Dunnings Mill is towards the end of the walk (olddunningsmill.co.uk)

A varied walk through the woodland and countryside south of East Grinstead.

① Take the footpath from the car park that heads south alongside the lane to Standen House. Immediately before it joins the road, turn right along a narrow path. When you arrive at a fork, bear left through a gate and continue downhill through a field until you reach another gate that takes you onto a path through woods. Continue straight on until you meet the Sussex Border Path, just before the Weir Wood Reservoir, where you turn left.

② Follow the Sussex Border Path as it follows alongside Weir Wood Reservoir for ¾ mile. Ignore a footpath turning to the left about halfway along this stretch. After ¾ mile the Sussex Border Path turns left, heading away from the reservoir. Follow this footpath, then bridleway, towards Busses Farm.

③ Just beyond the farm buildings, at a four-way fingerpost, go left through a gate into a field and follow the path through farmland in a westerly direction. When the path soon goes through a gap in the trees, turn immediately right and follow the tree line to a kissing gate. Go through the gate and follow the footpath through woodland, keeping to the main path straight ahead as you cross a bridge. When emerging from woods into a field, go diagonally right to a gate at the far side of the field. Go through the gate and continue straight on downhill until you eventually arrive at another junction before a stream.

4 Go immediately left, taking the footpath that follows the course of the stream. The path soon crosses another stream. Continue on with water to your right, walking until you reach Dunnings Road. Turn left at the road and walk a short distance to Coombe Hill Road.

5 Turn right into Coombe Hill Road and follow the road to a left turning into Medway Drive. Take this turn, which leads you on to the High Weald Landscape Trail. Continue for ½ mile until you reach a T-junction at a rugby field. Go left here and walk to the road. Once at the road cross over and take the path opposite leading you back to the car park.

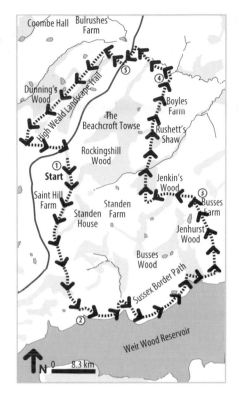

Points of interest

Standen House is an Arts and Crafts property built in the late nineteenth century and is considered to be one of the finest examples of its kind. The house and gardens are now owned by the National Trust and open for paying visitors.

Petworth Park

START Petworth Park National Trust car park, GU28 9LS, SU966240

DISTANCE 4 miles (6.4km)

SUMMARY A gentle, hilly route through the parkland surrounding Petworth House

PARKING National Trust pay and display car park (signed for the park not the house). Postcode: GU28 9LS

MAPS OS Explorer OL34; Landranger 187

WHERE TO EAT AND DRINK
Petworth House has a cafe but there is an entry fee, otherwise plenty of places to eat and drink in the town

This walk takes you all the way round the picturesque deer park surrounding Petworth House.

① Follow the path into the parkland with the wall on your right-hand side. It winds through trees and then leads along a wide path to reach a lodge. At the lodge, continue straight ahead uphill along the grassy path with the wall to your right. The path curves round a big old oak tree and leads fairly steeply up to a copse. Walk to the left of the copse, then continue straight ahead to reach a folly.

② At the T-junction by the folly go left, then turn right at the trees and follow the grassy path as it skirts the hill, taking in the staggering views as you go. The path winds its way under huge impressive trees and then forks. Take the right fork and walk towards the wall, then bear left and follow the path downhill towards a clearly defined track.

③ At the track, turn right. As you continue on, Petworth House begins to come into view. Ignore a left path leading to the seventeenth-century mansion and instead walk straight ahead towards a pond. Follow the path around the bottom edge of the large pond ignoring any turnings off it. This leads you around the water and then towards Petworth House.

④ Just before you reach some large black iron gates, bear left to follow the path leading past Petworth House (you can visit the house but must buy a ticket for entry).

5　Once past the house walk up the hill ahead of you. Follow the path straight ahead on the opposite side of the hill and as you walk, Lower Pond will come into view. Continue walking in the direction of the pond.

6　Continue straight ahead and follow the path, which takes you through the centre of the parkland designed by the famous Lancelot 'Capability' Brown, as it winds its way back to the car park. Keep your eyes peeled for deer as you walk.

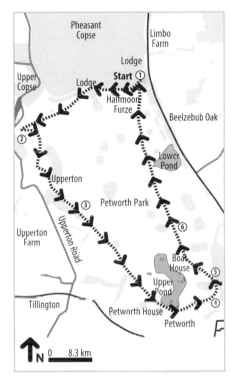

Points of interest

Petworth House in its present form with its sixty-three windows was built in the 1680s, although there has been a mansion house on the site since the early fourteenth century. Today Petworth is known for its extensive art collection, started by the third Earl of Egremont. The artist J. M. W. Turner was a frequent guest of the Earl and he painted views of the house and grounds.

Apuldram and Dell Quay

START Church of St Mary the Virgin, Apuldram, PO20 7EG, SU842031

DISTANCE 4 miles (6.1km)

SUMMARY An easy route along shoreline footpaths, lanes and roads

PARKING Free car park at the start point, PO20 7EG

MAPS OS Explorer OL08; Landranger 197

WHERE TO EAT AND DRINK The Crown and Anchor pub is close to the end of the walk (crownandanchorchichester.com)

A walk between Apuldram, Fishbourne and Dell Quay in Chichester Harbour, an Area of Outstanding Natural Beauty.

1️⃣ From the car park follow the signed footpath along a paved path towards the church. As soon as you enter the churchyard, turn left and follow the path along the bottom edge of the graveyard to a field. The path leads you along the edge of the field to reach the harbour side.

2️⃣ Turn right. At the next set of kissing gates take the left gate to remain on the harbour side footpath. At the following gate take the footpath straight ahead (the harbour side footpath is currently closed here due to erosion). When you reach the next gate go straight ahead then once over the sluice, go left to follow the shoreline again. The path soon crosses a footbridge and continues slightly inland alongside a wire fence.

3️⃣ Cross another footbridge then go right through a kissing gate and follow the path through the meadow. A boardwalk takes you into the next meadow. Ignore a gate on the right and the left in this field and instead continue straight ahead towards a building. Just before the building, when a path crosses yours, turn right and head to a gate into the churchyard. Once you've peeped inside the church, leave the churchyard via the main entrance by the car park and turn right going through a metal gate. Cross this meadow to reach a busy road. Turn right and then take the next road right signed for Apuldram.

4️⃣ Follow the road past houses. Just after the houses peter out, cross over and take the Salterns Way path on the left. Follow this clear path for around a mile. The Salterns Way runs relatively straight along the edge of fields and then bends right. Continue to follow the path until you reach a gate leading out to the road.

5. Continue in the same direction, then at the end of Apuldram Lane turn right. Follow this road (Dell Quay Road) straight ahead ignoring the Salterns Way turning on the left and another left-hand footpath further on. After just over ⅓ mile you will arrive at a waterside pub and Dell Quay.

6. Turn right and follow the shoreline footpath back to the turning for Apuldram church (point 2). From here retrace your steps back to the church and the car park.

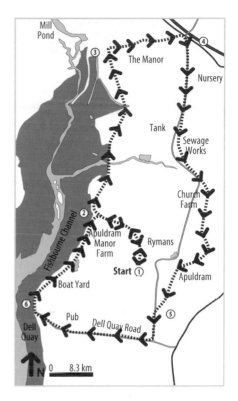

Points of interest

While it's now a peaceful hamlet with a waterside pub and sailing club, Dell Quay used to be a fairly major port serving nearby Chichester during medieval times.

Lancing Ring

START Lancing Ring nature reserve car park, BN15 0PX, TQ180063

DISTANCE 4¼ miles (6.8km)

SUMMARY A moderate route on byways, bridleways and footpaths; one steep climb

PARKING Free car park at Lancing Ring nature reserve. Postcode: BN15 0PX

MAPS OS Explorer OL11; Landranger 198

WHERE TO EAT AND DRINK None en route; selection of places to eat and drink in nearby Lancing

An elevated downland route offering stunning views over the surrounding coastline and the River Adur.

① From Lancing Ring car park take the main track leading away from the entrance road. Pass a metal gate and follow the byway, then when the path almost immediately forks go right. Follow the path ahead for 1¾ miles, ignoring any turnings off to the left. It leads you past the nature reserve and then up towards Steep Down where you walk around the right side of the hill. There are stunning views along this stretch of the walk.

② When you arrive at two sets of signposts, ignore the first junction then at the second four-way fingerpost turn right through a gate. Follow the bridleway along the top edge of the field with a hedgerow to your right and pylons down to your left. Continue for around 1 mile to reach a cattle grid by a copse.

③ At the cattle grid continue straight ahead to reach a second cattle grid. Once across continue walking with views of the sea ahead and follow the path as it veers to the right.

④ When you reach a three-way fingerpost close to the hamlet of Coombes, turn right through a gate and follow the footpath as it skirts the right-hand edge of the field. (To see Coombes church and village you can take a slight detour here by going straight ahead past the metal gate.)

Cross a stile and continue in the same direction. At a set of gates keep right and go through a kissing gate. The path leads gently downhill between hedges to reach another kissing gate. Cross a concrete farm track and follow the footpath leading straight ahead, downhill towards a stone cattle pen.

5 Once past the cattle pen (Cowbottom Hovel) go through a gate and begin the steep climb uphill. At the top go through the next kissing gate into open farmland. Keep straight ahead following the clearly defined footpath through the fields. Once across, pass through another kissing gate and continue ahead. A final kissing gate will take you to a T-junction where you turn right. The path almost immediately forks. Take the left footpath back to the car park.

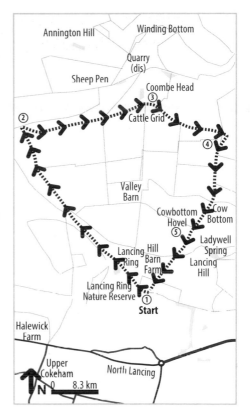

Points of interest

Coombes has an early medieval church that is well worth making a slight detour to visit at point 4 of the walk. The church contains twelfth-century wall paintings depicting the gospel story of the birth of Christ, which lay undiscovered until 1949.

Christ's Hospital

START Christ's Hospital rail station, Station Rd, RH13 0NE, TQ148292

DISTANCE 4¼ miles (6.7km)

SUMMARY A circular walk on bridleways, footpaths, lanes and road

PARKING Car park at Christ's Hospital rail station. Postcode: RH13 0NE

MAPS OS Explorer OL34; Landranger 198

WHERE TO EAT AND DRINK None en route

This circular walk starting at Christ's Hospital rail station takes you along the Downs Link and over to the pretty village of Itchingfield.

① Leaving the rail station car park, turn sharp left and follow the Downs Link in a northerly direction. This path leads you through a brick tunnel under the railway line and to some steps leading down into woodland. Descend the steps and follow the path alongside the river. The Arun springs from St Leonard's Forest to the east of Horsham and is just a stream at this point. The path winds through farmland and over a couple of footbridges following the riverbank.

② At a T-junction by a stone bridge turn left. Ignore a right-hand footpath and continue straight ahead. At a three-way sign by some gates, keep straight ahead to cross a bridge then continue along Mill Lane. Follow the quiet lane to a curved T-junction with another road then go right.

③ Follow Fulfords Road for just over 250yds, to where the road bends right (taking care as you go). Go left taking the quiet lane signed to Itchingfield. Follow the lane for almost ½ mile to reach the village.

④ Turn right to visit St Nicholas church. Enter the churchyard and take a path left which leads you around Priest House. Take the footpath out at the back of the churchyard and soon take a left bridleway across a field and head back to the lane.

⑤ Follow Fulfords Hill straight ahead with the old school to your right. Continue along the quiet lane until you meet a junction with another road.

[6] Turn right and soon take a footpath through a gate on the left. Follow the path along the edge of the field with trees initially to your left, then continue up to Sharpenhurst Hill where you get great views. Remain on the footpath as it descends and passes through a patch of woodland before arriving at the railway line. Cross the railway line with care, then cross a field and head down steps to reach the Downs Link path.

[7] Turn left and follow the path past Christ's Hospital school to reach Christ's Hospital Road. Continue ahead following the Downs Link along the pavement, keeping the railway line to your left. You pass a playing field on your right before arriving back at the station.

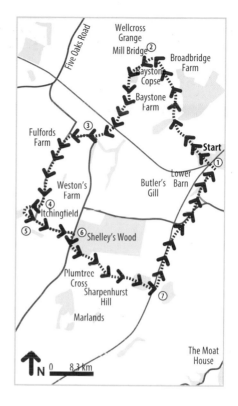

Points of interest

St Nicholas church in Itchingfield has a fifteenth-century timber-framed priest's house. The tiny building is thought to have been used for visiting monks and as an almshouse.

START National Trust
Lavington Common car park,
GU28 0QL, SU951184

DISTANCE 4½ miles (7.5km)

SUMMARY An easy walk along
footpaths and bridleways

PARKING National Trust car park
by the start. Postcode: GU28 0QL

MAPS OS Explorer OL10;
Landranger 197

WHERE TO EAT AND DRINK None
en route; the Foresters Arms pub
is in the nearby village of Graffham
(forestersarms-pub.co.uk/)

Explore Lavington Common on this peaceful walk through heathland and
woodland.

1 Leave the car park and take the footpath opposite. Follow it straight
ahead, ignoring a turning off to the right and another to the left. After
approximately ⅓ mile take a footpath on the right.

2 Follow the path down to a T-junction, then turn left. After around
100yds go through a gate and follow the left path along the edge of
woodland to reach a lane.

3 Go left at the lane and then after around 50yds take a right footpath
along an alleyway. When you reach a crossroads, keep straight ahead
and cross a meadow to another road. Turn left here and walk for around
50yds, then take a right-hand footpath leading between houses and then
bearing left. Continue down into woodland and cross a footbridge then
walk back up into a meadow where the path becomes indistinct. Go
straight ahead towards an oak tree and follow the path through a gate.
Continue across another meadow to the next gate and into woods.

4 At the fork go right. Walk for around 75yds to another junction and
take the right footpath. When the path forks again after a short distance
go left. Continue through woodland to reach a crossroads where you turn
right, then follow the bridleway for just over ¼ mile.

5 At the crossroads take the left footpath uphill. When you arrive at a
T-junction turn left and then go right following a footpath into Graffham

Common Nature Reserve. The path heads downhill and bears left before joining a bridleway. Go right and follow the bridleway to a lane.

6 Cross over and take the bridleway opposite. At the fork go left and walk past a farm. After around ¼ mile at a T-junction turn right onto a footpath. Walk past a barn and then turn immediately left continuing with a bank to your right. Follow this footpath for ½ mile as it winds its way through fields before running alongside a stream for a short distance and arriving at a lane.

7 Turn left and walk a short distance along the lane, then take a right-hand bridleway. When you get to a T-junction, turn right. The bridleway forks almost immediately, go left and follow it to where it bends round to the right. Leave the bridleway here and instead follow the track into heathland. When you arrive at a T-junction turn right and follow the footpath back to the car park.

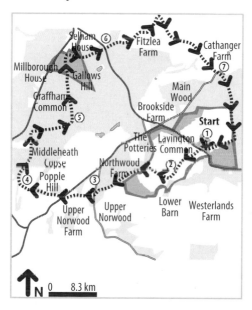

Points of interest

Lavington Common is a heathland nature reserve managed by the National Trust.

Hunston to Chichester

START Hunston Bridge car park, PO20 1NR, SU865023

DISTANCE 4½ miles (7.1km)

SUMMARY A moderate walk along footpaths, roads and canal towpath

PARKING Free car park at the start point. Postcode: PO20 1NR

MAPS OS Explorer OL08; Landranger 197

WHERE TO EAT AND DRINK Canal Cafe (chichestercanal.org.uk/canal-cafe) and a wide choice of other places to eat and drink in Chichester

A walk across fields to explore Chichester by foot before returning along the canal towpath.

① From the car park immediately turn right onto a public footpath leading through a gate and into fields. Follow this footpath through the meadow and along the edge of the next field to a footbridge. The path then passes bushes and paddocks to reach a quarry entrance. Cross this and take the footpath opposite through the gate. Walk to the end then cross the A27 using the huge footbridge.

② Once on the opposite side leave the bridge with the A27 on your left. Ignore the first right footpath, walking a short distance to another right footpath. Follow the alley to Sheffield Park Road and a housing estate. Cross the green, then take Exton Road to the left of the shops. Follow this round to a gap between houses where the road bends, then go right and soon right again along the alley to reach Kingsham Avenue. Turn left and cross over, then shortly go right along an alley to Stirling Road. Cross the railway line then follow Stirling Road straight ahead to a main road.

③ Cross and follow St John's Street opposite. Bear left towards a car park, then at Friary Lane turn right. Go left to follow East Pallant, then right at North Pallant walking past Pallant House Gallery to East Street. Go left here passing the Market Cross then straight ahead into West Street with the cathedral on your left.

④ At the end of West Street, turn left into Avenue de Chartres. Just past the restaurant on the corner take the entrance into Bishops Palace Gardens through the city wall. Follow the path winding through the gardens to a gate. Go left and follow the path leading out of another gate and then right to Canon Lane. Take St Richard's Walk left then go right at the cloisters. At the end, go right through a gate. This leads you past Vicars' Close and right past a row of cottages. At the end go left to reach South Street then turn right. Follow the road straight ahead to reach the railway line. Cross this then look out for Canal Wharf on the left.

5️⃣ Cross and turn into Canal Wharf then turn right past the pub and canal centre. Follow the towpath, with the canal to your left, back towards Hunston. Ignore any turnings off to the right and stick to the towpath for 1½ miles. At the bridge, cross over and make your way back to the car park.

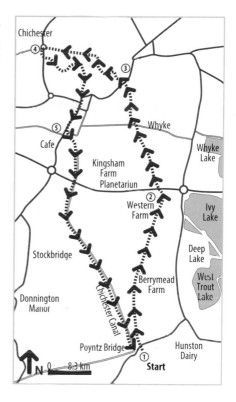

Bedham

START Wakestone Lane parking lay-by, RH20 1JR, TQ013220

DISTANCE 4½ miles (6km)

SUMMARY A moderate walk following footpaths, bridleways and short sections of lanes; can get muddy

PARKING Lay-by at the start. Postcode: RH20 1JR

MAPS OS Explorer OL10; Landranger 197

WHERE TO EAT AND DRINK None en route

A walk through ancient woodland around Bedham and past the ruins of an abandoned church.

① Start from the lay-by where Wakestone Lane bends sharply. Take the footpath signed for the Serpent Trail directly in front of the parking area.

Follow the path through the woods and past three large rocks. The trees begin to thin out and a field appears to your left. The path soon bears right and arrives at a crossroads.

② Go left and head uphill to reach a gate leading into fields where you get glorious views. Cross the field then climb a stile and head into the woods again. The path soon crosses a farm track where you continue straight ahead along a wide grassy path. Ignore a right turn and continue straight ahead with a field to your left.

As the path bends right, take a left footpath heading downhill alongside a brick wall. The path then climbs uphill to a T-junction – go left. Follow the path through the trees, then take the next signed footpath left.

③ Ignore a right footpath turning and continue ahead to cross a lane and climb a stile into a field. Follow the path diagonally left across the field heading under the pylon. Around ¾ of the way across the path bears right and heads towards the trees. Once back in the woods, head downhill to reach a lane. Go left.

④ Follow the lane uphill then shortly take a bridleway on the right. This leads down past the ruins of a church. Follow the bridleway to the right of the church leading downhill.

[5] At the T-junction take the left bridleway and walk through the woodland to reach a lane – go left.

[6] As you near the parking lay-by, take a right bridleway past a gate. Cross a track and continue straight ahead climbing steadily along the clear path, a section of the Serpent Trail. Remain straight ahead, ignoring any forestry tracks off to either side, for ¾ mile to reach a crossroads just before a road.

[7] Turn left. Follow the path through the woodland ignoring turnings off for ½ mile until you reach a cottage. Bear right and follow the drive to a lane.

[8] Turn left and follow the lane a short distance then take a left footpath back into the woods. Head straight uphill and continue through the woodland for just under ¾ mile until you arrive back at the start point.

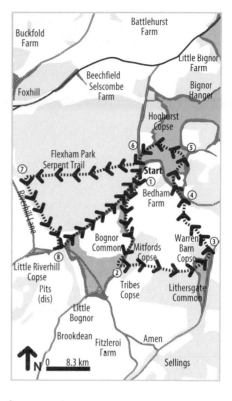

Points of interest

Bedham Chapel was built in 1880 and used as a school on weekdays and a church on weekends. The school shut in the early twentieth century and from 1959 there were no church services either. The building has been slowly decaying in the woodland ever since.

53 Storrington

START Our Lady of England Catholic church, RH20 4LW, TQ083141

DISTANCE 4½ miles (7.2km)

SUMMARY A moderate walk on bridleways, footpaths and lanes; one steep hill

PARKING Roadside parking by church. Postcode: PO18 0NJ

MAPS OS Explorer OL10; Landranger 197

WHERE TO EAT AND DRINK None en route

A simple route from the rural town of Storrington with a steep climb up to the South Downs Way.

1 From the Catholic church, take the public footpath which follows Kithurst Lane. The footpath then goes between driveways and heads along a narrow alleyway. Continue along the footpath until you reach a stile on the left, climb this and then follow the footpath to the next stile. Walk to reach Greyfriars Lane where you turn right.

2 Follow Greyfriars Lane past Gerston Farm and then after around 200yds, the road forks. Here, take the right-hand fork and head uphill where the road soon forks again at the next farm. Take the right-hand bridleway and follow it towards Coldharbour Cottage. When you get there, turn left.

3 Follow the bridleway to another fork in the path. Go left here and walk to a gate, then almost straight away turn right heading into the woods. Follow the bridleway as it curves to the left and climbs steeply up. At the top you will come to a crossroads with another bridleway. Follow the path running alongside a field and leading you to the South Downs Way.

4 Turn left onto the South Downs Way and follow it for almost a mile (ignoring a left-hand bridleway about halfway along) until you reach Kithurst Hill car park and Chantry Post.

5 Go left here, following Chantry Lane downhill for around 1 mile. About ¾ mile along the lane, just after you pass a pond, there is a small waterfall at the side of the road.

6 At a bend in the road, climb a stile on the left and follow the public footpath in a diagonal direction across fields. This footpath leads back to houses on the edge of Storrington. Walk left of the houses and then follow the signed public footpath straight ahead and then left into Brown's Lane. At Church Street, turn left again, then as you near the church turn right and follow the footpath back to the start point.

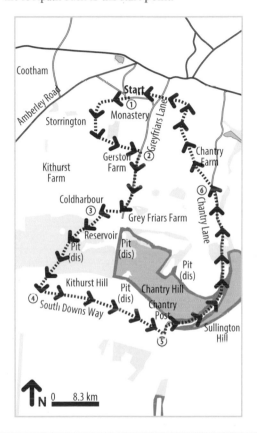

Points of interest

Storks have been making a comeback in Sussex in recent years after a successful re-introduction project at Knepp Wildland. But while you're unlikely to see any storks in Storrington today, the town was known as a hotspot for the elegant white birds in the past. In Saxon times its name was Estorchestone, which translates as 'homestead of the white storks'.

Pagham Harbour

START St Thomas a Becket Church, Pagham, PO21 4NU, SZ883974

DISTANCE 4½ miles (7.4km)

SUMMARY A moderate route on footpaths; the route must be completed at low tide – for tide times see www.metoffice.gov.uk/public/weather/tide-times/

PARKING Roadside parking on Church Lane. Postcode: PO21 4NU

MAPS OS Explorer OL08; Landranger 197

WHERE TO EAT AND DRINK Crab and Lobster at Sidlesham Quay (crab-lobster.co.uk)

An atmospheric walk packed full of birdlife around the RSPB Pagham Harbour nature reserve.

1   With your back to the church, turn right and walk to Church Farm caravan park. Go left into the holiday village and follow the footpath to a roundabout, then follow the sign for 'Lagoon Field'. After around 25yds leave the road and walk between caravans to a footpath. Turn right and follow the footpath around the edge of Pagham Lagoon with caravans to your right. At the end of the lagoon, follow the footpath right.

2   When the path forks, go left and follow the lower footpath along the edge of Pagham Harbour for just over ½ mile (when the tide is out).

3   When you reach the Salt House turn left and cross the sluice. Follow the raised footpath along Pagham Wall. Remain on this footpath for just over ½ mile, ignoring any footpaths going off to the right.

4   When the path forks by a three-way fingerpost, go right through a gate into a field. Follow the grassy path with the field boundary to your left. Ignore a footpath on the left by a gate and continue straight on along the left edge of the next field. Go through the kissing gate in the corner of the field and then follow the path between hedgerows to a stile. Turn left and follow the footpath along the drive, then out the gate and left onto Mill Lane.

5   Follow the lane for ¼ mile to reach the Crab and Lobster pub by Sidlesham Quay.

6 Turn left at the water's edge and follow the shoreline footpath as it twists and turns for almost 1 mile along the edge of the harbour (this section must only be completed at low tide). Ignore any footpaths going off to the left. A raised bank and some steps take you over the mud flats towards the end of this section.

7 When you arrive back at the three-way junction, go right and follow Pagham Wall back in the opposite direction to earlier. Walk past the sluice and Salt House, keeping straight ahead towards a paddock. The path bends right and meets Church Lane. Follow the lane for ¼ mile back to the church.

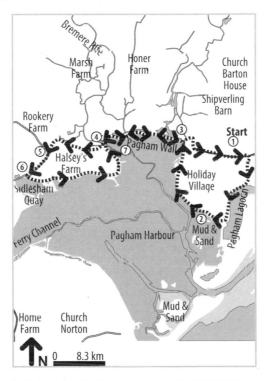

Points of interest

Pagham Harbour is rich in birdlife and a nationally important RSPB site for wintering ducks, geese and waders. In spring and summer you are likely to see little terns and egrets, which nest around the harbour.

55
56

Barnham

START St Mary the Virgin church, Barnham, PO22 0BP, SU955033

DISTANCE 4½ miles (7.3km) or 5¾ miles (9.2km)

SUMMARY Two easy walks following footpaths and lanes

PARKING Parking area near the church. Postcode: PO22 0BP

MAPS OS Explorer OL10; Landranger 197

WHERE TO EAT AND DRINK None en route

Two peaceful routes through the flatlands of Barnham and Yapton, visiting two hamlets along the way.

① From the parking bays, walk through the gate and follow the footpath ahead. At a crossroads by the site of an old canal swing bridge, turn left through a kissing gate and follow the footpath running along the long-defunct Portsmouth and Arundel canal. Follow this path straight ahead climbing stiles as you go. Ignore a left footpath turning and continue to a crossroads.

② Turn right taking the footpath through the field to reach two footbridges. Once across these continue across the next field. The footpath leads past paddocks and then joins a farm track. Walk past Drove Lane Farm to a T-junction with a lane.

③ a. For the short walk, turn right and follow Drove Lane for just under ½ mile through farmland, ignoring a left footpath turn, until you reach a solar farm. At the end of the track, bear left through a kissing gate and follow the path along the edge of the field, keeping the solar farm to your right to reach a fingerpost.
Go to point 6 to rejoin the longer route.

③ For the longer route, turn left and follow Drove Lane to a footpath turning on the right. Take this and head across the field, then bear left on the opposite side. At the next junction go right and cross the field to another footpath junction.

4 Turn right and continue straight ahead to reach Bilsham Lane, ignoring a footpath turning to the right and then the left as you walk.

5 At Bilsham Lane turn right. When the lane becomes a track continue straight ahead to reach a public footpath sign on the left. Follow the path across the field then bear left to cross a rife. Once across turn right and follow the footpath along the edge of the field to a solar farm. On the other side, turn left.

6 Continue ahead with the solar farm to your right. Cross a footbridge and go through a kissing gate, then continue straight ahead along the left side of a field to reach a gate. Follow the track ahead to a junction with another footpath.

7 Ignore the right footpath turning and head into the next field. The footpath runs through the middle of two fields to another junction by a gate. Turn left here and follow the footpath along the edge of the field to a stile and down to a lane. Turn right and walk past houses to a junction with another lane by a post box set into a flint wall.

8 Turn right and follow Hoe Lane through Flansham, ignoring any footpath turnings, until the road runs out and becomes a track. Follow this obvious track past a house and straight ahead. Ignore a left footpath and shortly after a right footpath, instead continue along the wide track.

9 When you arrive at a footbridge cross the rife, continue along the obvious track through farmland until you arrive back at the crossroads by the old swing bridge. Go straight ahead here back to the start point.

Iping and Chithurst

START St Mary's church, Iping,
GU29 0PE, SU852228

DISTANCE 4¾ miles (7.6km)

SUMMARY A moderate walk
along footpaths, bridleways and
lanes; one very steep climb

PARKING Roadside parking in
Iping. Postcode: GU29 0PE

MAPS OS Explorer OL33;
Landranger 197

WHERE TO EAT AND
DRINK None en route

A peaceful woodland route that passes through the grounds of a Buddhist monastery.

1 Follow the footpath leading through Iping churchyard and over a stile into a field. This leads you through fields and over a bridge crossing Hammer Stream. Continue through fields, then past farm buildings to a lane.

2 Take the footpath to the right of St Mary's Chithurst church, then follow it round to a stile leading into a large field with pylons. Go right following the edge of the field to reach another stile on the right. Descend the bank, turn left and walk to a T-junction where you turn right. Follow the restricted byway to a footpath on the left. This leads across a field, past a pylon, to reach a lane.

3 Turn right and walk approximately 150yds to a left-hand restricted byway entering woodland. Walk to a three-way fingerpost, then take the left footpath up a very steep hill. The scramble up is worth it for the views you get over the valley. Continue through the woods in this elevated position before a set of steps takes you up to a field leading to a road. Turn right and follow the quiet lane for approximately ½ mile.

4 When you reach a junction with another road go right, following the Serpent Trail along a lane towards Kinsham Farm. Just beyond the farmhouse go through a gate and continue straight ahead. The Serpent Trail soon goes off through a gate to the left, ignore this turning and continue straight ahead along the footpath. Climb a stile and walk diagonally across a field to some scrappy woodland, then wind through the next field and head up towards a cottage.

5 At the T-junction turn right and follow the restricted byway for approximately ¼ mile until you reach a gate on the left marked 'private woodland'.

6 Follow the permissive path through the peaceful woodland belonging to Chithurst Monastery. The wide path leads high up through Hammer Wood before descending steps to Hammer Pond. Soon, climb steps and walk around a house, then at the lane turn left.

7 Follow the lane before taking the next right footpath into a field. Skirt the edge of the field to a stile in the far corner, then follow the path diagonally across the next field to a kissing gate. Turn left, then at the lane go right heading back to Iping.

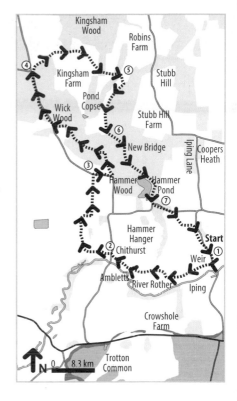

Points of interest

Much of the route is through the grounds of Chithurst Monastery, a Buddhist monastery founded in 1979.

Burton Mill Pond

START Car park by Burton Mill Pond, GU28 0JR, SU979180

DISTANCE 4¾ miles (7.5km)

SUMMARY An easy route along woodland and farmland footpaths and bridleways and quiet lanes

PARKING Small car park at the start point. Postcode: GU28 0JR

MAPS OS Explorer OL10; Landranger 197

WHERE TO EAT AND DRINK None en route; the Cricketers pub is in the nearby village of Duncton (thecricketersduncton.co.uk)

This interesting walk starts at an old hammer pond and then winds through peaceful countryside, woodland and heathland.

1   Walk to the road and turn right, then cross and take a footpath through gates for Burton Mill Lodge. Follow the drive then go through a gate into the Sussex Wildlife Trust Nature Reserve. Continue through woodland for almost ½ mile. Just past a grove of ancient sweet chestnut trees go through a gate and turn left onto a lane.

2   The footpath leads past houses then takes you over a bridge by a weir. Once past Chingford pond, the path bends left and heads into woodland. At the fork go right. Continue on for around 250yds to reach a road.

3   Continue ahead along the lane to reach a bridleway. Turn right and follow the bridleway through woodland to another lane.

4   Turn right following the lane until you see a sign for Keyzaston House, then take the bridleway leading along the right-hand side of a cottage. Stick to this bridleway (the Serpent Trail), ignoring another going off to the right after around 250yds. After around ⅓ mile you reach another lane.

5   Cross over and continue along the Serpent Trail, which leads through a gate into Lord's Piece and Sutton Common. Walk straight ahead over the heathland and when the path forks, go left walking uphill towards trees. The route can become a little unclear through this section but keep to the bridleway ignoring any paths off it and you should pass a white building

on your right (an old school house), before going through a gate to reach a lane.

⑥ Turn right and walk for just over ⅓ mile until you reach a church. Not far past the church there is a footpath on the left. Take this past the house.

⑦ Follow the signed footpath across farmland to a crossroads. Go straight ahead with a field to your left and woodland to your right. After around ⅓ mile a farm track forks off to the left, ignore this and bear right following the footpath downhill to woodland. Walk through the woods then climb a stile and continue up to a T-junction. Go left and walk through a field to a lane.

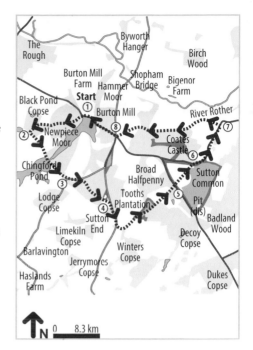

⑧ Turn right and follow the lane downhill (signed to Duncton). This leads you back to Burton Mill Pond.

Points of interest

Burton Mill Pond is an old hammer pond, a relic of the iron-making industry in Elizabethan England. Today it's a nature reserve and home to dragonflies, beetles, bitterns and warblers.

START Parham Park entrance on Rackham Street, RH20 2EU, TQ049143

DISTANCE 4¾ miles (7.6km)

SUMMARY An easy route along footpaths, bridleways and lanes; one footpath crosses an airfield

PARKING Limited roadside parking on Rackham Street. Postcode: RH20 2EU

MAPS OS Explorer OL10; Landranger 197

WHERE TO EAT AND DRINK None en route

A varied and interesting circular walk through the parkland of Parham House and surrounding farmland and woodland.

1 Go through the white gates into Parham Park and follow the broad public footpath (Sussex Literary Trail) straight ahead. The path takes you past a lake and Parham House and soon after to a T-junction. Follow the signed footpath straight ahead as it leads gently uphill through the deer park.

Follow the footpath as it curves round and then follows the line of a road passing an eighteenth-century ice house on the right. Keep going until you get to the park gates.

2 Leave the park and turn right at the road. Walk for around 50yds, then cross over and take the left footpath towards Southdown Gliding Club. Walk a short distance then turn left again towards cottages, then right and over a stile. This footpath winds round to reach Parham Airfield and then leads you straight across it. Once across the airfield take the footpath left and follow it as it winds through farmland before leading into the woods. Keep straight ahead through the woodland, ignoring a footpath to the left, until you reach a lane.

3 Turn left at the lane, walk a few paces, then follow the surfaced bridleway on the right. After around ⅓ mile a footpath goes off to the right, ignore this and continue along the bridleway with a fence on your left. The sandy bridleway leads through woodland for another ⅓ mile before arriving at a main road.

4 Cross the road and take the signed bridleway on the opposite side into Wiggonholt Common. Walk through the woodland a short distance to reach another road. Cross over and continue on the bridleway opposite. Follow the

signed bridleway through mixed sandy woodland for ¼ mile to a junction with a footpath leading up to Pulborough Brooks RSPB reserve. Ignore this turning and continue straight ahead on the bridleway to reach a road.

⑤ Cross the road and continue ahead along the quiet lane on the opposite side. Follow the lane through the woodland for just under 1 mile until you arrive back at the gates for Parham House and Gardens.

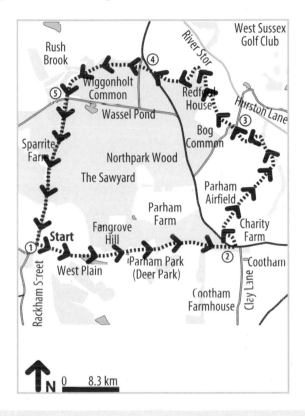

Points of interest

Parham House and Gardens is a sixteenth-century mansion house which Queen Elizabeth I is said to have visited. It was built following the Dissolution of the Monasteries by Henry VIII. Having fallen into disrepair, the house was restored in the 1920s and 30s by its new owners and has been open to the public since the 1940s.

Arun Valley 1

START Arundel rail station, BN18 9PH, TQ024063

DISTANCE 5 miles (8km)

SUMMARY A moderate riverside walk along footpaths, bridleways and lanes and a short section of busy road

PARKING Rail station car park by the start point. Postcode: BN18 9PH

MAPS OS Explorer OL10; Landranger 197

WHERE TO EAT AND DRINK The Black Rabbit is midway along the route (theblackrabbitarundel.co.uk/); the Bridge Inn is close to the end point (bridgeinnamberley.com/)

A riverside walk between Arundel and Amberley rail stations through the beautiful Arun valley.

1　From Arundel station, head towards the town. Once in Arundel, cross the bridge over the River Arun and turn right into Mill Road. Almost immediately turn into Jubilee Gardens and cross to the far right corner of the small park, heading behind the museum to join the riverside footpath.

2　Stick to this footpath for almost 2 miles as it follows the course of the meandering Arun, ignoring any turnings off to the left. There are fantastic views back over to the town, the castle and the surrounding South Downs countryside along this stretch.

3　When you reach the car park and Black Rabbit pub, leave the riverside and follow the lane leading uphill behind the pub. At the top of the hill at a T-junction with another lane turn left and shortly after take the right-hand bridleway leading downhill. Once the path flattens out, walk to reach a gate then keep straight ahead to cross a field via a fairly indistinct path. The bridleway crosses a drainage ditch and continues to reach another gate on the opposite side. Continue straight ahead until you reach the tiny hamlet of South Stoke.

4　At the lane turn right and follow it round to the church. Take the path to the left of the church that leads down to a bridge crossing the Arun, then once across take the footpath on the left. The footpath follows the banks of the river for a short distance, then heads into a patch of damp woodland and soon reaches a suspension bridge. Cross the bridge and then continue on to reach a kissing gate. The footpath crosses a field and soon arrives at a road in the next hamlet of North Stoke.

⑤ Turn left onto the lane, then soon after turn right to follow Stoke Road downhill. Ignore a bridleway turning off to the right soon after and then a footpath on the left after around 300yds (this footpath can be very overgrown). Continue along the road, walking past the Bridge Inn, then turn right at the main road and head under the railway bridge. Amberley rail station can be found shortly on the right with regular trains running back to Arundel.

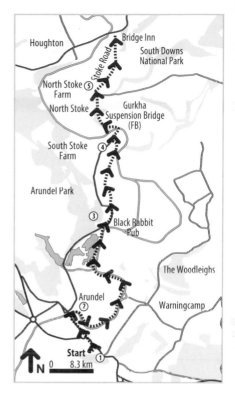

100 Walks In West Sussex   117

Points of interest

The hamlets of South Stoke and North Stoke are referenced in the Domesday Book and both have medieval churches that are well worth a visit.

Knepp Wildland

START Shipley Windmill, RH13 8PL, TQ143219

DISTANCE 5 miles (8km)

SUMMARY An easy-going walk following footpaths, bridleways and lanes

PARKING Parking bays on School Lane. Postcode: RH13 8PL

MAPS OS Explorer OL34; Landranger 198

WHERE TO EAT AND DRINK None en route; the Countryman Inn is close by (countrymanshipley.co.uk)

A beautiful walk through the varied landscape and restored habitats of the Knepp Wildland Project.

①   With your back to the windmill go right and follow School Lane as it curves to the left and meets Red Lane. Shortly after crossing Kings Platt, take the footpath on the right, which runs behind houses and heads into a small patch of woodland. Walk straight ahead through the trees ignoring any permissive paths off either side. Cross a field and then at the road go left for a few paces, then cross and turn right onto the footpath opposite.

②   Enter Knepp Wildland and follow the broad path through the parkland. At the drive turn right, then when a second drive meets from the left take the broad grassy footpath on the right. When the path meets another drive, turn right. The footpath follows a lane. Just before Trollards Barn take the footpath on the right.

③   The path leads to long footbridges (over the Adur) and then to a gate. Go through the gate and turn left following the footpath to another gate, past a house and out to a road. Turn right and follow Swallows Lane to where it meets Countryman Lane, then take the left footpath leading down a private road.

④   Follow the road down to a gate to reach a pond. Turn left and follow the clear footpath to where it forks, go right.

⑤   Continue straight ahead ignoring any turnings off either side until a signed footpath forks off to the left leading you under mature oaks and alongside a ditch. When you emerge from the trees, cross the path and follow the grassy footpath almost directly opposite. This leads to a gate, go through and then turn right at the T-junction.

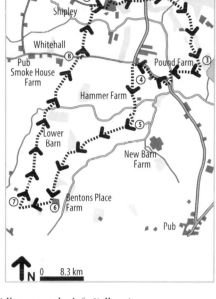

6 Follow the footpath through the trees ignoring turnings to the right and left. Instead keep straight ahead to reach a T-junction.

7 Go right and follow the bridleway through a gate and to a crossroads. Keep straight following the clear bridleway ahead for around a mile. Ignore a left footpath turning as you go and continue straight on to reach a lane.

8 Turn right and walk approximately 40yds, then take the bridleway on the left. Follow it through the trees and across a bridge. The bridleway passes the windmill and leads back to School Lane. Turn right to return to the parking bays.

Points of interest

In 2001 the Knepp Estate was transformed from a farm to a re-wilding project with free-roaming animals grazing the land. As a result very rare species such as purple emperor butterflies, nightingales and storks are making a comeback.

Wolstonbury Hill

START Jack and Jill Windmills
car park, BN6 9PG, TQ302134

DISTANCE 5 miles (8km)

SUMMARY A moderate hilly route
on bridleways, footpaths and lanes,
with two small sections along
pavement beside a main road

PARKING Free car park at start
point. Postcode: BN6 9PG

MAPS OS Explorer OL11;
Landranger 198

WHERE TO EAT AND DRINK
The Coffee Mill, a horse box cafe
serving food and drink by the
windmills is open at weekends
and some weekdays during
the summer (m.facebook.
com/thecoffeemillclayton)

An interesting hilly downland route on the border with East Sussex, offering
amazing and far-reaching views.

1   From the main car park entrance turn left and follow the bridleway
up the lane leading gently uphill. You soon arrive at the South Downs Way
where the path forks. Bear left following the path uphill. At the top take
the right-hand bridleway off the South Downs Way and follow it as it leads
back downhill to a crossroads by a farm.

2   At the crossroads walk straight ahead rejoining the South Downs
Way leading downhill past a golf course. Go through the golf club car park
and down to a main road. Cross over and turn left remaining on the South
Downs Way running beside the road to reach School Lane.

3   Turn right into School Lane. Just before the church turn right
following the bridleway along The Wyshe. Once past cottages and a play
park, continue steadily uphill. At the first crossroads continue straight
ahead then at the next crossroads turn left.

4   Follow the bridleway through a gate into Wolstonbury Hill (National
Trust). Terrific views immediately open out. After around ¼ mile, go
through a gate and walk to the fingerpost ahead. Take the right footpath
and follow it up to the trig point at the top of the hill.

5 Follow the grassy open access path to the right of the trig point leading down with a view of the windmills ahead. Continue straight on towards a gate at the bottom of the hill. At the ladder stile continue straight ahead.

6 Go through the gate and turn left, following the footpath that winds downhill through the trees. When the path forks, bear right walking past a house with a large chimney and down a drive to a lane. Turn right and follow the lane to a main road ignoring a footpath on the left and a bridleway on the right as you go.

7 Turn right and cross the railway bridge, then cross the busy road to take Underhill Lane opposite. Walk past Clayton church then take the next bridleway on the right, heading up to the South Downs Way.

New Way Lane
Ockenden's Wood
Garden Centre
Butcher's Wood
Bonny's Wood
Lag Wood
Hautboyes
Coldharbour Farm
Halfway
Little Danny
The Warenne
7
Clayton
5
Wolstonbury Hill
6
Pit (dis)
8
Clayton Holt
4 Rockrose
Jill
Jack
Chantry
Clayton Tunnel
1 Start
New Barn Farm
Wayfield Farm
3
South Downs Way
2
Haresdean
Rag Bottom
Middle Brow
Pangdean Cottage
Pangdean Farm

↑ N   0   8.3 km

8 Go through a gate and take the second left-hand footpath leading uphill. The footpath loops round and rejoins the bridleway. Follow this path fairly steeply back up to the windmills.

Points of interest

It's well worth popping into St John the Baptist church in Clayton on the way past to see the medieval wall paintings adorning the walls of the small Anglo-Saxon building.

Graffham

START St Giles church, Graffham,
GU28 0NJ, SU928167

DISTANCE 5 miles (8km)

SUMMARY A moderate hilly
walk along footpaths, bridleways
and restricted byways

PARKING Roadside parking by the
start point. Postcode: GU28 0NJ

MAPS OS Explorer OL10;
Landranger 197

WHERE TO EAT AND DRINK
None en route; the White Horse
is in nearby Graffham village
(whitehorsegraffham.com)

A gorgeous walk taking in woodland, farmland, open downland and a stretch of
the South Downs Way.

1   With your back to the church, turn right and walk along the road
heading towards Graffham Down. Once at the end of the road continue
in the same direction along the restricted byway, ignoring a footpath
turning off to the right after a short distance. When you get to a staggered
crossroads take the restricted byway left, and remain on this undulating
path through woodland for ½ mile.

2   When the path forks go left and head downhill, keeping straight
ahead when you come to a crossroads with a footpath. The byway leads
past Seaford College and then splits. Continue straight ahead and walk
uphill to reach a T-junction where you turn sharp right. Follow the
bridleway uphill for around ⅓ mile to a junction with a footpath, then
turn left. Continue climbing uphill and you will soon emerge from the
woods. Bear left and follow the footpath diagonally towards the South
Downs Way and once there, turn right.

3   Follow the path to a crossroads where you go straight ahead and then
remain on the South Downs Way, ignoring any turnings off either side
to reach another crossroads leading to an entrance into Graffham Down
Trust Reserve. If you fancy exploring the reserve, head for this gate, but to
continue on the route, remain on the South Downs Way, continuing ahead
for almost ¾ mile until you reach a restricted byway turning on the right.

④ Take this right turn and begin the descent down Graffham Down. Remain on the byway ignoring a footpath turning to the left and another footpath which crosses the byway soon after. When another byway turns to the right, ignore this and continue on to a T-junction.

⑤ Go right and follow the footpath steeply up. When you reach a fork in the path go left. Follow this undulating footpath as it weaves its way through the woodland for just over ⅓ mile. When you arrive at a crossroads turn left and head steeply down. Once down a set of steps, turn left and walk back to the church.

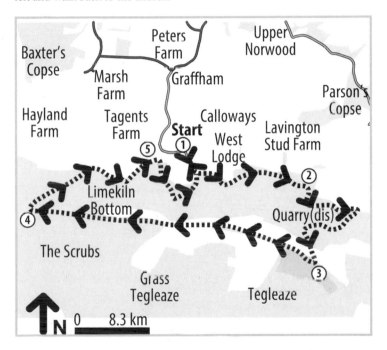

Points of interest

The Graffham Down Trust Nature Reserve, which you can explore with a short detour off the South Downs Way, is an environmental project aiming to protect areas of open downland and its indigenous flora and fauna. The conservation work undertaken since the 1980s has led to more varieties of wildflowers and butterflies, with animals such as dormice making a comeback too.

Ouse Valley Viaduct

START Ardingly Reservoir car park, RH17 6SQ, TQ335286

DISTANCE 5 miles (8.1km)

SUMMARY The route follows footpaths, bridleways and lanes

PARKING Large car park at the start point. Postcode: RH17 6SQ

MAPS OS Explorer 135; Landranger 198

WHERE TO EAT AND DRINK None en route

A circular route from Ardingly Reservoir to the huge Victorian-built Ouse Valley Viaduct.

1 From the car park walk up to the reservoir and turn left. Pass a boatyard and go straight ahead, walking up to a kissing gate into woods. When the footpath forks keep left and enter a field via a gate. Cross the field, then climb the stile and cross the next field where you should get your first glimpse of the Ouse viaduct on the left. Cross the next stile and another field bearing slight left towards a lane.

Follow the path with a large country house to your right (Balcombe Place). The tarmac path then bears left by farm buildings and leads down to a main road.

2 Cross over and take the footpath opposite. The path goes over a footbridge and continues to a bridge over the railway line. Once across turn right and walk alongside the railway before heading downhill with woodland on your right. Ignore a right turn into the woodland, instead keeping straight ahead to reach a stile. Cross the field to a bridge, then follow the footpath to reach a road.

3 Cross over and take the bridleway opposite. Keep straight ahead until you pass a farm and then follow the drive down to a lane. Turn left and follow the lane for ½ mile to reach a main road.

4 Go left for a few paces then cross and take the footpath opposite along a farm track. You are now following the Sussex Ouse Valley Way, a 42-mile long-distance footpath that follows the route of the River Ouse. Just before the farmhouse take the footpath left through a gate and down steps. Walk along the raised bank with a hedgerow to your right. The path

leads across a footbridge and stile, then veers right across a field. Continue through fields until you reach the next farm.

⑤　Walk through the farm and follow the drive round to the left, then take the footpath on the right towards the viaduct. Once under, cross the next field to the road.

⑥　Turn right and follow the road over the Ouse then immediately take a footpath left. When you reach a footbridge, cross the river and walk through the field to the next footbridge. Head uphill until you see a gap in the hedgerow on the right, then take this path leading back to the reservoir.

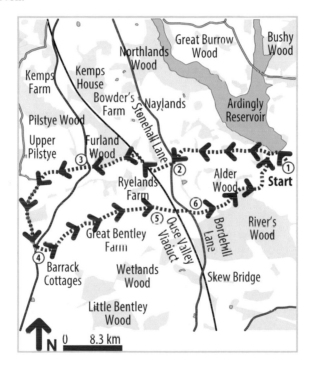

Points of interest

The Ouse Valley Viaduct was opened in 1841. It's a hugely impressive 96ft-high structure made up of thirty-seven brick arches and is over ¼ mile long.

Chidham

START Cobnor Farm amenity car park, PO18 8TD, SU791037

DISTANCE 5 miles (8km)

SUMMARY An easy walk on footpaths, shingle and quiet lanes; the beach section at Cobnor Point is inaccessible during high tide, so tide tables much be checked prior to walk (www.metoffice.gov. uk/public/weather/tide-times)

PARKING Free car park (small). Postcode: PO18 8TD

MAPS OS Explorer OL8; Landranger 197

WHERE TO EAT AND DRINK The Old House at Home, Chidham, is close to the end of the route (theoldhouseathome.co.uk)

A beautiful coastal walk around Chichester Harbour at Chidham and Cobnor Point.

1. Leave the car park via a small set of steps and turn left onto a private road. Follow this for a short distance to a fingerpost then turn left and follow the footpath along the edge of a field towards the Bosham Channel where you turn right. Walk along the raised bank with the water to your left admiring the views over to Bosham, until you arrive at a Christian Youth Enterprise Centre.

2. At the centre, fork right heading downhill and around to the right. Cross the lane and a footbridge then follow the footpath straight ahead through an avenue of trees. The footpath leads around a house and a small boatyard before winding left back to the water's edge and onto a wheelchair accessible path. Follow this path to some steps leading down to the beach.

3. THIS SECTION FLOODS AT HIGH TIDE.
Walk along the shingle beach passing some weather-beaten oak trees and a bird hide along the shoreline. Climb a set of steps and continue along a raised bank, enjoying more fine views across Nutbourne Marsh Nature Reserve and Nutbourne Channel to your left. When the path forks by a noticeboard go right and continue on until you reach a fence.

4 At the fence continue along the footpath onto the sea wall and then after a short distance take a sharp right down some steps. Continue along the bottom edge of the field, walking back on yourself in the direction you just came from. The footpath soon follows the edge of the field around to the left and heads inland. When you arrive at a footbridge, cross it and continue straight ahead with trees on one side and hedgerow on the other.

5 At the lane turn right and walk to a fingerpost, then turn left and follow the footpath into a field. Follow the footpath with the church spire ahead of you, then turn right at the next fingerpost. When you reach the lane keep straight ahead. At the T-junction turn left and follow the lane back to the car park and the start point of the walk.

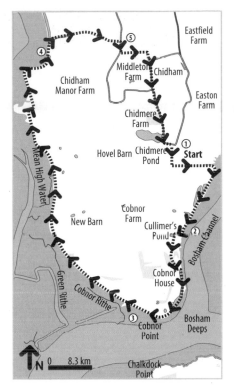

Middleton Farm   Chidham

Chidham Manor Farm

Easton Farm

Chidmere Farm

Mean High Water

Hovel Barn   Chidmere Pond   **Start** ①

②

Bosham Channel

Cobnor Farm

New Barn

Cullimer's Pond

Green Rithe

Cobnor Rithe

Cobnor House

Bosham Deeps

③ Cobnor Point

N   0   8.3 km

Chalkdock Point

Points of interest

Nutbourne Marsh Nature Reserve is home to a variety of birds such as oyster catchers, egrets and curlews, which feed on the exposed mud flats at low tide. Seals can sometimes be spotted around Cobnor Point.

Milland

START The Rising Sun pub, Milland, GU30 7NA, SU838269

DISTANCE 5¼ miles (8.3km)

SUMMARY An easy route along footpaths, bridleways, lanes and road

PARKING Roadside parking close to the start point. Postcode: GU30 7NA

MAPS OS Explorer OL33; Landranger 186

WHERE TO EAT AND DRINK
The Rising Sun pub is at the start and end of the walk (www.risingsunmilland.com)

An interesting walk through the farmland and woodland surrounding the village of Milland.

1. Starting with your back to the pub and facing a four-way road sign, turn right to follow the road signed for Linch. Continue past a pond and go left when the road forks. Ignore a left footpath and soon after take a right bridleway through a gate and along a gravel path. Go through the next gate and continue past houses to a T-junction. Go left. Follow the bridleway past cottages to your right to reach a gate. Follow the bridleway through a patch of woods and on to a lane.

2. Turn left and follow the lane to where it bends right, then take a footpath left. At a crossroads continue straight ahead over the stile and across the field. Climb the next stile into woodland. Follow the footpath through the woods, bearing right when it forks. The paths weaves up through the woodland and when you emerge there are fantastic views. Climb a stile and follow the path along the left edge of a large field, then cross another stile and continue alongside the left of the next field. At the crossroads by gates take the bridleway right.

3. Follow the bridleway gently downhill, bearing left when it forks by a large barn, to reach a junction by a drive. Here take the footpath straight ahead along the drive.

4. At the crossroads turn left onto the restricted byway. Ignore a left turn into Forestry Commission woods and continue to a left bridleway. Follow this through the woods and along the edge of a golf course. At the T-junction go right. The bridleway leads along the top of the golf course

and then splits. Bear left. The bridleway soon swings right and then forks left to reach a road.

5 Turn left and follow the lane through the stone pillars (taking care as the lane is narrow). Pass Milland House (ignoring turnings either side) then take a left-hand bridleway forking off from the road. Follow the track down past a large house to reach a T junction.

6 Turn left and follow the bridleway a short distance then take a footpath right. When the path forks, bear left and continue on as it winds through the trees to a crossroads. Go right and walk to reach a gate.

7 Once through the gate turn right then almost immediately bear left, following a narrow path to another gate. Follow the footpath diagonally right across the field, then cross the next field to an old mill. Cross an L-shaped footbridge, then climb steps and follow the drive ahead to the road.

Turn left and head back to Milland.

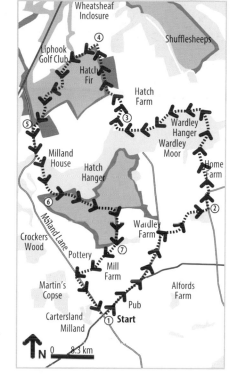

Points of interest

Milland Mill and mill pond date from the late seventeenth or early eighteenth century and are associated with the area's iron-making industry.

Walderton to Stansted House

START Breakneck Lane, Walderton, PO18 9ED, SU787104

DISTANCE 5¼ miles (8.4km)

SUMMARY An easy walk along footpaths, bridleways and lanes

PARKING Lay-by parking by the start. Postcode: PO18 9ED

MAPS OS Explorer OL08; Landranger 197

WHERE TO EAT AND DRINK
The Barley Mow pub is close to the start (thebarleymow.pub)

A varied walk through farmland and woodland taking in Stansted House and the ruins of a folly.

1 From Breakneck Lane walk back to the main road and turn right. After around 100yds when the road bends right take a small road (Woodlands Lane) leading off to the left and follow the bridleway along it. Continue along the lane for just over 1 mile, walking through woodland and ignoring a bridleway turning on the right.

2 When you reach a junction by a gate, ignore any turnings off to the left and right and instead continue straight ahead. Follow the bridleway for a little over ½ mile to reach a tree-lined lane.

3 Go left at the lane and walk past the gates to Stansted House. Just past here, turn left to follow a bridle path signed for the house. This takes you past the imposing house and grounds and soon arrives at a road. Bear right and follow the road for around 50yds, then turn left onto a footpath.

4 Follow the path past the tea room to reach a zebra crossing, then turn left to walk through a patch of woodland. You soon arrive at a gate – go left and walk across the field. On the other side of the field go through a gate and continue along the footpath to a kissing gate where you turn left. Walk a few paces to a crossroad junction by a stile.

5 Take the restricted byway ahead with fields to your right. Follow this path ignoring any turnings off to the left or right for around 1½ miles

until you reach a main road. The byway takes you through woodland and past the ruins of an eighteenth-century folly (the Racton Monument).

[6] Once at the road turn left and walk for approximately 200yds to reach a footpath turning on the left. Climb a stile into a field and then follow the footpath diagonally across to a house. Cross the drive to a footpath that follows the course of a stream and then follow it past Lordington House to a stile. Continue across the farmland until you arrive at houses and a road. Turn right onto the lane, then right again at the main road and retrace your steps back to the start point of the walk.

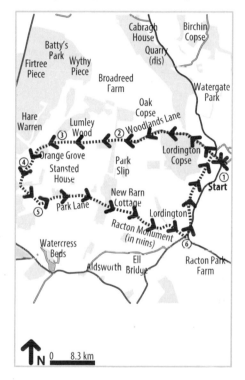

Arundel Water Woods

START Chalk Springs Fishery, Park Bottom, Arundel BN18 9HD, TQ012069

DISTANCE 5¼ miles (8.5km)

SUMMARY A moderate route along bridleways, footpaths open access land; one fairly steep climb

PARKING Roadside parking in Arundel. Postcode: BN18 9HD

MAPS OS Explorer OL10; Landranger 197

WHERE TO EAT AND DRINK None en route; plenty of cafes, pubs and restaurants in Arundel

A woodland walk starting by a fishery on the site of old watercress beds on the edge of Arundel.

1   Enter Chalk Spring Fisheries via the entrance between gatehouses off the A27 and follow the bridleway on the left heading uphill. When you reach the top, the bridleway bends to the right while a footpath goes straight ahead. Ignore the footpath over the stile and remain on the bridleway, ignoring any turnings off it, for just over ½ mile until you eventually reach a gate on the left.

2   Follow the bridleway through the gate into a field. Go through the next gate and walk with the hedgerow to your left over to another gate. Continue along the bridleway, ignoring a footpath on the left until you reach some woodland.

3   At the woods, the track forks. Follow the bridleway right into the woodland. Go through a gate and continue straight ahead, then cross a wide forestry track. Keep straight ahead walking for a further ¼ mile to where the bridleway forks.

4   At the fork follow the bridleway to the right. When the path forks again, bear left and soon head steeply downhill. Go through a gate into an open access area and continue straight ahead on the bridleway for a short distance until you reach a crossroads. Go right here to follow a grassy path through the nature reserve for around ⅓ mile to reach a gate, then continue through the woods. At the fork, take the path on the right and keep walking until you reach a grassy area close to the road.

5 Turn right onto the public footpath and climb the steps taking you up the steep hill. Follow the signed footpath, bearing left as another path forks off it and go through a gate. The footpath joins and then crosses a forestry track, then heads downhill. At the bottom of the hill, cross a track and keep straight ahead, following a narrow footpath up through the scrub and then under large yews. Remain on the signed footpath for just under a mile as it winds up and down through the woods, and then alongside fields, ignoring any forestry tracks criss-crossing the path as you go.

6 As you approach a main road take a footpath on the right. Follow it downhill to a crossroads, then go left following the restricted byway towards buildings. Walk through a small group of office buildings and workshops then continue along the road. Continue straight ahead, ignoring two footpath turnings into the woods as you go. This byway takes you past the fishery on the left and back to the start point.

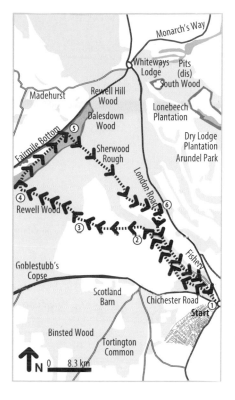

Points of interest

The large trout fishery you walk past towards the end of the route was created in the 1980s out of old Victorian watercress beds.

Kingley Vale

START The Hare and Hounds
pub, Wildham Lane, Stoughton
PO18 9JQ, SU803115

DISTANCE 5⅓ miles (9km)

SUMMARY A moderate hilly walk
along footpaths, bridleways and lanes

PARKING Roadside parking by the
start point. Postcode: PO18 9JQ

MAPS OS Explorer OL08;
Landranger 197

WHERE TO EAT AND DRINK The
Hare and Hounds pub is at the start
and end point (02392 631433)

A walk offering fabulous views, a grove of ancient yew trees and some Bronze Age
burial mounds.

① Starting with the pub to your left, walk along Wildham Lane
towards Old Bartons cottages and take the footpath right (the Monarch's
Way). Walk past a barn then bear left and continue through farmland.
After around ¾ mile the footpath is joined by a left-hand bridleway.
Keep straight ahead following the bridleway as it begins to climb up to
Stoughton Down and soon heads towards woodland.

② When you arrive at a crossroads turn right and follow the bridleway
along the edge of woodland. After around ⅓ mile, when the path forks, go
left and walk to reach a crossroads by a Kingley Vale noticeboard.

③ At this crossroads turn right and follow the bridleway through
woodland, then head up to reach an area of open downland.

④ Turn sharp left at the Devil's Humps, taking a path directly opposite
the burial mounds leading downhill to reach a gate into Kingley Vale
Nature Reserve. Take the lower path straight ahead into yew woodland.
When the path forks go right and head steeply downhill. Continue along
this path until it forks again where you go right, following the broad path
through the trees and out to the valley.

⑤ The path leads you down past a pond. From just beyond the pond
follow a path on the left to reach a group of huge ancient yew trees. Just
past the grove you will arrive at a T-junction. Turn left and follow the path

for approximately ⅓ mile. It heads
back into woodland and passes
a visitor centre on the left before
reaching gates.

⑥ Turn right onto the bridleway
and walk for around 100yds to
another bridleway turning. Take
this right as it leads uphill to reach
another entrance into Kingley Vale
Nature Reserve where the path
forks. Go left, continuing to follow
the bridleway as it climbs through
farmland and then heads into
woods. After around ¼ mile when
the path forks, go right.

⑦ Follow the bridleway uphill
ignoring two right bridleway
turnings as you walk. Once back in
woodland it heads steeply downhill.
Remain on the clear path as it leads
back to Stoughton for ¾ mile.
When you arrive at the lane, turn
right and follow it back to the pub.

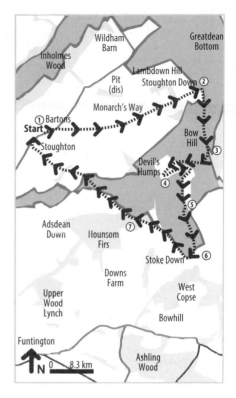

Points of interest

The Devil's Humps near point 4 of the route are Bronze Age burial
mounds. You also pass a grove of yew trees (point 5) that are thought
to be around 1,000 years old, some of the oldest trees in Britain.

Centurion Way

START Centurion Way, Westgate, Chichester, PO19 3HR, SU848047

DISTANCE 5½ miles (9km) one way from Chichester to West Dean or 11 miles (18km) return

SUMMARY An easy and accessible route ideal for wheelchair users or parents with buggies

PARKING Roadside parking close to the start point. Postcode: PO19 3HR

MAPS OS Explorer OL8; Landranger 197

WHERE TO EAT AND DRINK The Selsey Arms at West Dean (selseyarms-westdean.co.uk) or West Dean Stores (westdeanstores.co.uk)

An accessible path following the route of a disused railway line between Chichester and West Dean.

① Begin the walk from the start point of the Centurion Way, which is clearly signposted close to Bishop Luffa School. The beauty of this walk is that most of it is an easy straight route with lots of interesting points along the way. The shared user path runs along the old Chichester to Midhurst railway line, which was closed in 1991. It's since been surfaced meaning users can easily walk or cycle and people who can't ordinarily access the countryside easily – wheelchair users or parents with prams – can do so here. Follow the path straight ahead passing the school to your right. Ignore any footpath turnings on either side as you walk.

② After just under 1½ miles you will come to Brandy Hole Copse Nature Reserve on the left. It's worth a quick detour into this nature reserve to explore its history and wildlife (however there are no surfaced paths so it wouldn't be suitable for everyone). The mature woodland is blanketed by bluebells in late spring and there are World War Two anti-tank defences as well as Iron Age earthworks to be found. Once back on the Centurion Way, continue in the direction of East Dean.

③ Approximately ½ mile further along you will arrive at some metal sculptures, 'The Chichester Road Gang'. At a bridge the path forks – go straight ahead, under the bridge and continue in the direction of Lavant and West Dean.

④　When you arrive at a residential area continue straight ahead passing a playground on the right. Keep walking straight through the housing estate (following Churchmead Close, then Springfield Close) and when you reach a green, cross it diagonally bearing right. You then arrive at the next clear section of the Centurion Way. Follow the surfaced path for approximately 2 miles enjoying the views as you go.

⑤　When you arrive at West Dean tunnel you can access the village via a set of steps or a ramp. The shorter route ends here and there are regular bus services (number 60) from West Dean taking you back to Chichester. Alternatively for a longer route, simply retrace your steps back along the Centurion Way to Chichester.

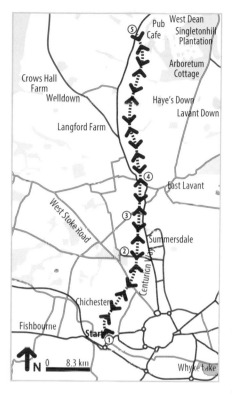

Points of interest

'The Chichester Road Gang' – a set of sculptures created out of empty oxygen gas cylinders by artist, David Kemp. The group of figures marks the spot where an old Roman road to Silchester crosses the Centurion Way. The Roman road lay undiscovered until the 1940s.

Bignor Hill

START Whiteways Lodge car park, BN18 9FD, TQ001108

DISTANCE 5½ miles (8.7km)

SUMMARY An easy route mainly along woodland and farmland bridleways

PARKING Free car park at the start point. Postcode: BN18 9FD

MAPS OS Explorer OL10; Landranger 197

WHERE TO EAT AND DRINK Whiteways cafe in the car park at the start point

A woodland and downland walk along a stretch of the South Downs Way offering spectacular views from Bignor Hill.

1 Starting from the Whiteways car park with your back to the main road, follow a bridleway past metal gates and enter into the woodland. When the path soon forks bear left and continue along the signed bridleway as it leads you through the beech and conifer woodland of Houghton Forest for around ¾ mile.

2 When you arrive at a T-junction by a clearing, turn right and follow this bridleway (the Denture), continuing through the woodland and ignoring any turnings off the bridleway on either side for around 1¼ miles.

3 When you arrive at a crossroads by a tree-trunk bench, turn right and follow the bridleway up towards Bignor Hill car park. Once there, go right again, heading in the direction of the road and then follow the South Downs Way right, steadily climbing up to Bignor Hill, where, on a clear day, you can enjoy fantastic far-reaching views over the surrounding countryside and out to sea. Remain on the South Downs Way following it round a field and then turning left and leading downhill.

4 Once down the steep hill go right and walk to the crossroads where you continue straight ahead along the South Downs Way for just over 1 mile. When the path forks with a track on the left, continue straight ahead following the South Downs Way through the fields to reach a crossroads with a bridleway.

⑤ At the crossroads go right, leaving the South Downs Way, and following the bridleway downhill to a field. Walk through the field with the hedgerow to your left and then enter woodland. Follow the grassy bridleway for around ½ mile until you reach a junction with lots of paths shooting off. Take the first left-hand bridleway here, which leads you back to the Whiteways car park, the start and end point of the walk.

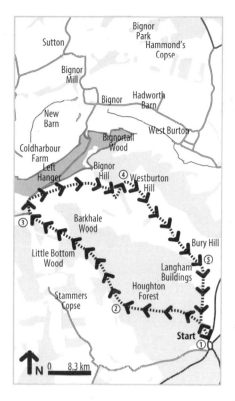

Points of interest

At the car park on top of Bignor Hill you will see a signpost pointing in the direction of Londinium (London) to the north and Noviomagus (Chichester) to the south. In Roman times, Stane Street ran through here connecting the two cities via the 57-mile-long road. Further evidence of Roman life can be found in the nearby village of Bignor, where there are the remains of a substantial Roman villa.

START Finches Field public car park, Church Hill, West Hoathly, RH19 4PN, TQ367325

DISTANCE 5½ miles (8.7km)

SUMMARY A moderate walk following footpaths, bridleways and lanes

PARKING Finches Field car park at the start. Postcode: RH19 4PN

MAPS OS Explorer 135; Landranger 187

WHERE TO EAT AND DRINK The Cat Inn is at the start and end point (catinn.co.uk/the-pub)

An interesting and varied walk featuring the Bluebell Railway, a reservoir and a sandstone crag.

① From the car park follow a footpath past some allotments. Descend steps to the road, cross and take the footpath opposite. The footpath soon meets a bridleway – continue straight ahead downhill to reach Bluebell Lane. At the end of Bluebell Lane turn left to follow the Sussex Border Path along a private drive. The drive eventually turns right, passing under the Bluebell Railway line.

② Once under the railway line, climb a stile and continue along the track past New Coombe Farm. Shortly after, take an enclosed path straight ahead leading into woodland. Continue ahead, crossing a stream, then immediately turn left following the path uphill to reach a junction. Turn left, taking a narrow path between fields to a road.

③ At Grinstead Lane, turn left, walk a few paces, then take the right footpath which shortly joins a road. Continue to the school, then take a footpath straight ahead to reach the Weir Wood reservoir. At the lane turn left and follow it alongside the reservoir until you meet another road.

④ Turn right and cross the bridge, then follow the road uphill for just over 300yds. Ignore Admiral's Bridge Lane shooting off to the right and soon after take a bridleway on the left. Continue for around ¼ mile to where the path forks, looking out for the Stone Farm Rocks SSSI along the way.

⑤ At the fork, go right, remaining on the bridleway and walking past woodland on your right. Ignore a left-hand footpath turning and continue for nearly 300yds past a stream and a pond. Just past the pond ignore a right bridleway turning and continue ahead, walking through a farm and back to the railway line.

6   Once over the railway go right at the fork following the bridleway through the trees. Ignore a left footpath and continue along the bridleway as it swings to the right, soon joining a road that loosely follows the line of the Bluebell Railway and then heads uphill through woodland.

7   Just after crossing a stream take a left footpath and follow it for around 150yds. At a crossroads follow the High Weald Landscape Trail left down to a river crossing. After crossing, fork right and head uphill to a road. Continue past a farm and at the top of a hill, turn left along a metalled road. Follow this to Gravetye Manor, then take the footpath to the left of the gates, going downhill and over a stream. Go through a kissing gate and follow the path as it winds up through trees. At the top you will arrive at a track. Turn right and continue uphill, through a kissing gate, and then straight on.

8   When you reach houses follow the drive to the road. Cross over and take North Lane opposite, then follow it for around 450yds past a school. Just before a church, turn left into Church Hill and return to the car park.

Points of interest

Stone Farm Rocks (point 4) is a sandstone crag and a geological Site of Special Scientific Interest (SSSI).

St Leonard's Forest

START Roosthole car park, St Leonard's Forest, RH13 6PG, TQ210295

DISTANCE 5½ miles (9km)

SUMMARY A moderate walk mainly on woodland and farmland footpaths and bridleways; plenty of stiles

PARKING Free car park at the start point. Postcode: RH13 6PG

MAPS OS Explorer OL34; Landranger 198

WHERE TO EAT AND DRINK None en route

An interesting walk in St Leonard's Forest and surrounding countryside, part of the High Weald Area of Outstanding Natural Beauty.

① Take the broad track leading away from the car park and head into the forest. When you reach a T-junction (Mick's Cross) go left.

② Follow the straight wide track ahead ignoring any forestry tracks off the main path. At a four-way fingerpost go right. Another path soon forks off to the right, ignore this and continue straight ahead and downhill.

③ Once downhill, turn left and walk a short distance to where two paths go off to the right. Take the first footpath and head downhill to a stile. Continue straight ahead.
   Just before you reach a cottage, go right through a gate and walk between fences to a field. Climb a stile and cross the field (keeping left), to a set of stiles. Ignore a left footpath and continue straight ahead through the next field and over another stile, then cross a stream.

④ Continue through woods to reach a three-way fingerpost by the corner of a field. Go straight on here to reach a lane.

⑤ Cross over and take the footpath opposite leading to a gate. Skirt the left side of the field to reach another lane. Turn left.

⑥ Follow the lane past houses until you see a footpath on the right. Follow this down into woodland and continue with a fence to your left. The path then swings to the right and descends to a stream, then climbs up to a gate entering a field. Follow the path along the left edge of the field and head uphill to reach a farm.

⑦ At the crossroads turn right and follow the bridleway for approximately ½ mile along the lane, enjoying views over the valley as you go. As the lane heads down and curves to the left, turn right onto a bridleway.

⑧ Ignore a right footpath turning and continue ahead on the High Weald Landscape Trail to reach a gate. Go through and head into trees, then cross a footbridge and follow the chalky bridleway as it swings left into open grassland. At the T-junction go right and walk up to a road.

⑨ Cross over and take the footpath opposite. The path leads down to a stream, then winds gently up through the woodland for almost ½ mile to reach a junction. Follow the High Weald Landscape Trail sign left for a short distance back to Mick's Cross, then go left and almost immediately right to follow the unsigned track back to the car park.

Holmbush Forest
Beacon Hill
High Wood
Rookfield Farm
Colgate
Black Hill
Woodside Farm
Knights Strength
Blackhouse Farm
Forest Grange
St Leonard's Forest
Newstead Ghyll
Whitevane Pond ③
④
⑥
⑤
Greenbroom Hill
Barnsnap Wood
Elenge Plat Farm ⑦
Scragged Oak Hill
② Grouselands Farm
Tattleton's Farm
① Start
The Goldings
⑨
⑧
Old Copse
Grouse Road
Carter's Lodge

N 0   8.3 km

Points of interest

According to legend, sixth-century hermit St Leonard lived in the forest where he fought and killed the last dragon in England.

Sutton

START St John the Baptist church, RH20 1PX, SU979154

DISTANCE 5½ miles (8.7km)

SUMMARY A moderate walk along footpaths, bridleways and quiet lanes in the South Downs National Park; some steep hills

PARKING Free on-street parking outside the church. Postcode: RH20 1PX

MAPS OS Explorer OL10; Landranger 197

WHERE TO EAT AND DRINK The White Horse Inn (whitehorseinn-sutton.co.uk)

A circular walk from the pretty village of Sutton up to the South Downs for stunning countryside views.

1   With the church to your right, walk for around 50yds to a right-hand bridleway. Take this and continue up to where the path forks, then go right again. Follow the bridleway round and then along the edge of a field. When you reach a directional cross-post in the centre of the filed, take the left footpath. Cross the field, then continue on, walking between houses to reach a road.

2   At the road, pass the pub (White Horse Inn) and take the lane right. Turn immediately left onto a footpath and follow it uphill past a cottage. Cross the field and continue down to a patch of woodland. Go through a gate, then follow the path as it bears right, and winds its way through the trees and over a stream to reach a lane.

3   At the lane turn right and shortly after take the right-hand footpath. When the path forks, go left and follow the edge of the field. Continue along the left of the next field walking towards hills. Go through a kissing gate and then head steeply uphill towards woodland. Cross the bridleway and continue up the Downs until you reach another lane.

4   Turn right and continue climbing uphill to reach a National Trust car park. From here continue straight on along a wide bridleway through gates, ignoring any left turns. This leads uphill towards large radio masts and through more gates. Walk past the masts then continue straight ahead through gates before heading downhill.

5 Once at the bottom of the field go through gates then continue steeply downhill. The bridleway bears right and leads into woodland, then almost immediately forks. At the fork go left. Follow the bridleway between hedges and up to a gate. Go through and continue for around 200yds to reach a set of gates leading into a field. Continue down through the field to reach a crossroads at the bottom.

6 At the crossroads, go straight ahead then almost immediately go right. Follow the footpath down through woodland (this path does get steep).

7 Once at the bottom of the hill, cross the field towards a barn. This takes you to a lane. Cross over and take the bridleway opposite into a field. Follow this bridleway straight ahead and when you reach a crossroads maintain direction and retrace your steps back to Sutton and the church.

Barlavington Hanger
Jerrymores Copse
① Start
Haslands Farm
Northcomb Wood ⑦
Folly Lane
Sutton
②
Court Farm
Bignor Mill
⑥
③
Farm Wood
Glatting Farm
New Barn Farm
Glatting Lane
Pitchurst Copse
Coldharbour Farm
⑤
Left Hanger ④
Glatting Beacon
Bignor Hill
Monarch's Way
Gumber Corner
Barkhale Wood
N   0   8.3 km
Great Bottom

Points of interest

St John the Baptist parish church at the start of the route. The oldest parts date from the eleventh century with substantial additions made in the fourteenth century.

Amberley

START Amberley rail station,
BN18 9LR, TQ026118

DISTANCE 5½ miles (8.9km)

SUMMARY A moderate hilly
walk mainly along bridleways,
byways and lanes

PARKING Parking by the start
point. Postcode: BN18 9LR

MAPS OS Explorer OL10;
Landranger 197

WHERE TO EAT AND DRINK
The Bridge Inn, Amberley is
close to the start and end point
(bridgeinnamberley.com)

A downland walk along mainly mud-free paths with magnificent views and some
Neolithic earthworks to admire.

1   From the railway station entrance turn left and walk out to the main
road. Cross over and go left again at the main road, and walk under the
railway bridge, then just past the pub, take the lane on the left (Stoke
Road) signed for North Stoke. Follow the lane, ignoring a footpath
turning to the right and a bridleway turning to the left as you go. The lane
eventually leads up and round to a T-junction with another lane. Turn left.

2   Follow this lane, ignoring a bridleway turning to the right, for just
over 1 mile as it leads gradually uphill. When you arrive at a gate, where
the lane ends and the path forks, go left.

3   Follow the restricted byway and head uphill for just over ¼ mile
to reach a crossroads. Keep straight ahead here and continue along the
byway for another ¼ mile until you arrive at a T-junction. Turn left again.

4   Follow this byway for just over ¾ mile until you reach another
junction.

5   Just after a bridleway joins from the right, take the byway left and
continue along up towards the South Downs Way. When the path forks
shortly afterwards bear right and continue on to reach some small hills at
the end of the path.

6 These two small hills are in fact Neolithic earthworks, and make for the perfect spot to stop and enjoy the atmosphere and views. After stopping, turn left onto the South Downs Way and begin heading steadily downhill. There are more impressive views to enjoy along here.

7 Once at the bottom of the hill, when you reach the next junction, continue walking along the South Downs Way. The path leads through a small patch of woodland to reach a quiet lane. The South Downs Way then continues right along the lane (High Titten). When the road soon forks, go left.

8 Follow the lane downhill to reach the main road. Turn left and cross over to follow the path alongside the road, leading back to Amberley rail station.

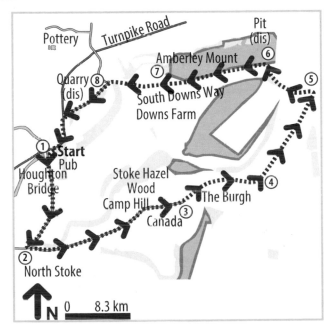

Points of interest

The small hills found at point 6 of the route are ancient earthworks dating from the Neolithic period and are believed to have been boundary markers.

Rudgwick and Rowhook circular

START Rudgwick Chapel,
Rudgwick, RH12 3EE, TQ090341

DISTANCE 5½ miles (9km)

SUMMARY A moderate walk following
footpaths, bridleways and lanes

PARKING Windacres Farm Lane
(opposite Rudgwick Chapel), RH12 3EE

MAPS OS Explorer OL34;
Landranger 187

WHERE TO EAT AND DRINK The
Kings Head pub is close to the
start and end point of the walk
(kingsheadrudgwick.co.uk) or
the Chequers Inn in Rowhook
(thechequersrowhook.com)

A peaceful walk between the villages of Rudgwick and Rowhook on the border
with Surrey.

① From Rudgwick Chapel, walk south along Church Street, then just
before you reach Summerfold, take the signed footpath left along the
path that runs parallel to the road. Follow this as it wiggles its way to
meet another footpath at a bridge, then take the left fork and head uphill.
The footpath continues for another couple of hundred yards to meet a
crossroads with a bridleway. Remain straight ahead here and walk on
through the woods until you meet another footpath.

② Go right and then very shortly after fork right again. This footpath
leads you past Hyes and then down to some ponds (the site of an old
ironworks). Continue through the woods and past the ponds until you
reach the gates to Furnace Lakes Estates.

③ Turn left immediately and take the path leading into Roman Woods.
Follow this path as it winds through the trees, ignoring any forestry tracks
off either side for ¾ mile until you reach a fingerpost showing a right turn.
Turn right and follow the path to reach a T-junction.

④ Turn right and follow the bridleway through the woods ignoring
any turnings on either side until you come to Waterlands Lane at Burnt
House. Turn left and follow the lane along past the Chequers Inn.

⑤ After approximately 200yds, just as the road bends left, take the left
footpath over a stile. Follow the footpath uphill through a field. At the top,

go straight across another field to the right-hand corner and cross a small bridge. Emerging from the trees, go diagonally right past Millfield House and then through a gap in the trees ahead. Turn immediately left, passing a pond on the left before heading into woodland. Cross a footbridge in the woods and continue on past a reservoir to reach a T-junction.

6 Turn right onto the metalled road. When you reach a farm, turn left onto the Sussex Border Path and follow it for approximately ¾ mile. Ignore a footpath turning off to the left and the right, continuing straight to reach a lane.

7 Cross over and take a bridleway opposite. When the bridleway meets a crossroads, go right along a narrow path, continuing along the Sussex Border Path. This leads you back to the village of Rudgwick, past the church. When you join the road, turn left and walk back to the Rudgwick Chapel.

Points of interest

The ponds passed at point 2 on this walk are on the site of an Elizabethan ironworks.

Angmering Park Estate

START Dover Lane car park,
BN18 9PX, TQ060061

DISTANCE 5½ miles (8.9km)

SUMMARY A moderate
walk mainly along woodland
footpaths and bridleways

PARKING Free car park by the
start. Postcode: BN18 9PX

MAPS OS Explorer OL10;
Landranger 197

WHERE TO EAT AND
DRINK None en route

A peaceful circular walk through the bluebell woodland of Angmering Park Estate.

1   From the car park turn right onto Dover Lane, then at the crossroads go straight ahead taking the bridleway leading towards fields. Follow the path as it swings left and walk to a cottage. The path turns to the right here, follow it for around ¼ mile to a footpath turning on the left.

2   Take the left footpath leading up into the woods (the woodland floor is smothered in bluebells through here in late spring). Follow this path for just over ½ mile, keeping straight ahead at a crossroads until you reach a lane.

3   Cross the lane and then turn almost immediately right onto the first bridleway. Remain on this bridleway as it leads you gradually uphill with views opening out to the left as you go. After approximately ½ mile there is a footpath turning on the left – ignore this and continue on for just over ½ mile more. The bridleway then crosses an open grassy area to a gate into open downland. Walk uphill across the field with a fence to your right. The bridleway follows the line of the fence as it bends to the right and leads to gates.

4   Once through the gates take the bridleway leading diagonally left. Cross a farm track and head down to another gate, then follow the bridleway in and out of woodland for almost a mile to a T-junction with another bridleway.

5   Go right and follow the bridleway through the woods until you reach a footpath turning on the left.

6 Follow the footpath, which joins a wide path after around 100yds and then passes stables and paddocks. Once past a large house you arrive at a T-junction. Take the footpath left and then shortly after turn right walking past a pond. The path continues uphill for just over 200yds to a gate by a crossroads with another footpath. Remain straight ahead here and cross the field to the woods.

7 Enter the woods and then turn right onto a bridleway. Remain on this bridleway for ½ mile, keeping straight ahead at a crossroads, until you arrive back at the start point of the walk.

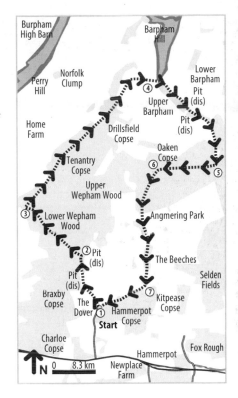

Points of interest

Angmering Park Estate forms part of the Duke of Norfolk Estate with its origins dating back to the Norman Conquest. Today it is used for farming and sporting purposes and is blanketed with bluebells each year in spring.

Henley

START Duke of Cumberland pub, GU27 3HQ, SU894257

DISTANCE 5¾ miles (9km)

SUMMARY A moderate route along bridleways, footpaths, byways and lanes; some steep climbs

PARKING Roadside parking by the pub. Postcode: GU27 3HQ

MAPS OS Explorer OL33; Landranger 197

WHERE TO EAT AND DRINK Duke of Cumberland Arms at start/end point (dukeofcumberland.com)

A peaceful figure-of-eight woodland walk through Verdley Wood and Bexleyhill Common.

① Take the Serpent Trail footpath opposite the pub past a phone box. Shortly after, turn left and walk between houses, over a footbridge and into woodland.

After approximately ¼ mile you reach a junction with forestry tracks where the broad path narrows and continues through trees. Keep to the footpath for nearly 1 mile ignoring the multitude of forestry tracks criss-crossing the path. If in doubt look for the purple Serpent Trail markers, which are well signed throughout. Ignore a left bridleway turn as you go and continue to a lane.

② Cross over and take the footpath opposite leading up and around the hill. At the top the footpath curves round to the left before the ground levels out. When you arrive at a three-way junction continue ahead along the broad path. At a crossroads with a forestry track continue straight ahead again. When the path forks go right to follow the elevated path to reach a crossroads by an old barn.

③ Go left following the bridleway downhill, ignoring a left turn shortly after. At the next crossroads take the left bridleway, heading downhill past a pylon. Fork left at the bottom of the hill and follow the narrow path winding uphill. At the top follow the bridleway ahead to reach a three-way junction.

④ Take the bridleway straight ahead ignoring a left forestry track. You are now back on the Serpent Trail. Once past some cottages, ignore a right bridleway turning. Follow the Serpent Trail along the lane and then turn left heading to the road.

⑤ Go left and walk into Bexleyhill. This leads back to the point where you left the Serpent Trail earlier. Take the restricted byway right heading into Verdley Wood walking for around ¾ mile to reach Surney Farm. Walk ahead along the lane for a few paces then take the left footpath.

⑥ The footpath leads between fences and winds uphill back into woodland. Cross a couple of footbridges then climb back up and follow a wide grassy footpath that soon swings to the right. When the path forks, go right.

⑦ At a T-junction go right and follow the bridleway for around 100yds. Take a left footpath and follow it for ⅓ mile to a T-junction by a cottage. Go left following the byway past the cottage to the road. Turn left, heading back to the pub.

Points of interest

According to legend the last wild bear in England was killed in Verdley Wood. What is known is that during medieval times there was a hunting lodge in Verdley Wood called Verdley Castle.

Warninglid

START The Street, Warninglid,
RH17 5TT, TQ249260

DISTANCE 5¾ miles (9km)

SUMMARY An easy route along
footpaths, bridleways and lanes. Can
be muddy in parts after wet weather

PARKING Roadside parking in
Warninglid. Postcode: RH17 5TT

MAPS OS Explorer OL34;
Landranger 187

WHERE TO EAT AND DRINK The
Half Moon pub in Warninglid
(thehalfmoonwarninglid.co.uk)

A circular walk through wooded valleys and countryside surrounding the High
Weald village of Warninglid.

① Start from The Street in Warninglid, walking in a southerly direction,
past houses and away from the village. As the road bends to the right, take
the path straight ahead towards Routwood Farm. The path soon forks left
and follows a lane leading through fields.

At the farm take the bridleway left walking past barns and then
through fields. Pass a pond and go through a metal gate, then continue on
towards a house. Follow the bridleway along the drive to the road.

② At the road, turn right and head downhill. As the road bends take a
footpath on the left. Follow the footpath uphill through two kissing gates,
then into woodland and continue on, enjoying the views, until you reach a
driveway where you turn right.

③ The drive leads to a crossroads. Go straight ahead and then shortly
take a path leading right running past two houses. Follow this bridleway
for around ¾ mile to reach a road.

④ Turn left at the road and walk for approximately 100yds to a footpath
on the right. Walk downhill to reach a T-junction then go right. After
around 100yds the bridleway forks – take the right-hand footpath into
woodland and continue downhill until you arrive at another junction with
a bridleway.

⑤ Turn right here and follow the bridleway past a pond and through a
small field to a crossroads where you turn right again. When you arrive

at the junction with Mill Lane continue along the bridleway, which leads you through woodland to a large pond and then back into the woods. When you arrive at a small bridge follow the path as it turns left. Walk along the wooded valley keeping to the bridleway for approximately ¾ mile to reach a crossroads.

6 Keep straight ahead at the crossroads walking uphill and sticking to the signposted bridleway. The path soon bends and drops down to cross a brook before climbing back up again and then heads to a road. Turn right and follow the road for ⅓ mile back to Warninglid (you will need to walk along the verge for a short section along this stretch). When you reach The Street turn right to arrive back at the start point of the walk.

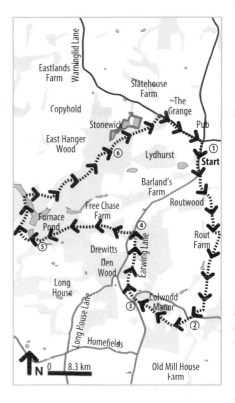

Points of interest

Wealden House, which you pass along The Street at the start of the walk, is believed to have been lived in by the poet Tennyson for a short time in 1850. He and his wife fled after a storm blew down their bedroom wall.

Burpham and Wepham Down

START The George at Burpham, BN18 9RR, TQ039089

DISTANCE 6 miles (10km)

SUMMARY A moderate walk following footpaths, bridleways and lanes; some parts can be muddy

PARKING Free car park by the start point. Postcode: BN18 9RR

MAPS OS Explorer OL10; Landranger 197

WHERE TO EAT AND DRINK The George at Burpham is at the start and end point (georgeatburpham.co.uk)

A walk from Burpham in the South Downs National Park with beautiful views over the Arun valley.

1 From the pub turn left and follow the road a short distance, then almost immediately take the next road right. Follow the lane past houses with the church on your right to reach Peppering Farm. At the farm go right and continue along the lane for around ¼ mile to where the road splits.

2 Go right and follow the lane downhill for another ¼ mile. At the crossroads keep straight ahead and then shortly afterwards take the bridleway on the left.

3 Follow the bridleway for just under ¾ mile, passing through a gate as you go. Continue straight ahead to reach a fork in the path.

4 Here take the right-hand footpath leading uphill. Once at the top climb the stile and follow the footpath through the field to reach a T-junction. Turn left and follow the broad footpath that leads you round to another junction.

5 Take the bridleway left to reach gates. Go through the gate and follow the bridleway left heading downhill.

6 Continue along the bridleway as it rises and falls for 1 mile, ignoring any turnings off the main path. There are far-reaching downland views to enjoy as you walk this stretch. Continue on until you get to a T-junction.

7 When you reach the T-junction, go left. Follow this bridleway for a short distance then take the grassy bridleway on the right. Ignore a turning on the right and follow the bridleway, which soon becomes chalky underfoot. Continue straight ahead for approximately ⅓ mile until you reach a footpath on the right by a gate.

8 Turn right and follow the footpath downhill. Climb a stile and descend the steps then go left to follow the path along the edge of the meadow. Keep straight ahead ignoring a right turning. The footpath leads to a stile on the right into a field, then to another stile followed by another two fields. Follow the signed footpath to reach the banks of the River Arun.

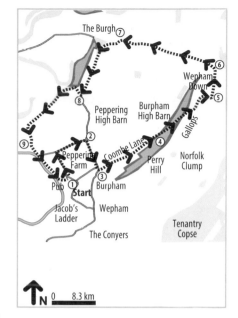

9 Continue along the footpath with the river to your right. Go through a gate then right through another gate. Follow the path across the meadow then through another gate and uphill. When you reach an alley turn left and follow it to reach a lane, then follow the road back to the pub.

Points of interest

Mervyn Peake, artist and author of *Gormenghast* lived in the area from the 1930s and is buried in St Mary's church graveyard.

Charlton and Levin Down

START The Fox Goes Free pub, Charlton, PO18 oHU, SU887129

DISTANCE 6 miles (9.6km)

SUMMARY A moderate hilly walk along woodland and farmland footpaths and bridleways

PARKING Roadside parking. Postcode: PO18 oHU

MAPS OS Explorer OLo8; Landranger 197

WHERE TO EAT AND DRINK The Fox Goes Free pub at the start/ end point (thefoxgoesfree.com)

A hilly walk through varied and interesting South Downs countryside, including a nature reserve.

① Follow Charlton Road for around 100yds towards Singleton and go right following the West Sussex Literary Trail along North Lane. The bridleway heads uphill, past a farm and eventually forks.

② At the fork, go right past a gate and up steps. The footpath (still the West Sussex Literary Trail) bears right and continues climbing as it crosses a field to the corner. Continue on to a turning on the right, then follow the wide path for around 100yds where it turns left and through a kissing gate. Cross another field, then climb a stile and enter woodland.

③ You soon arrive at a crossroads. Turn left and remain on this footpath through the woods and past a field for approximately 350yds, ignoring any forestry tracks as you go. When you get to a crossroads with a bridleway, keep straight ahead. Remain on the footpath for just over ½ mile through the woodland until you arrive at a large junction with multiple paths.

④ Go right, following the signed footpath leading uphill through the woods. Continue on this footpath for ½ mile, ignoring any forestry tracks, until you reach the South Downs Way.

⑤ Turn left onto the South Downs Way and follow it for ¼ mile. Continue ahead at the crossroads, then at the second crossroads turn left.

⑥ Follow the footpath for around 150yds to a junction with a bridleway, then turn right. Follow the bridleway downhill through the woodland for just under a mile, ignoring any forestry tracks off either side. As you emerge from the woods follow the bridleway along the left-hand side of a field and continue bearing left when the path forks. You soon reach a crossroads where you take the bridleway right, the New Lipchis Way.

7 The path leads through a gate and along the right-hand side of a field. Walk uphill and go through a gate. The bridleway soon bears right, then heads downhill to reach another junction.

8 Turn left onto the footpath. When you arrive at a T-junction go left, heading uphill. This leads to gates into Levin Down Nature Reserve. Follow the footpath through the reserve, enjoying the views as you go. The path winds down to reach a field leading back to Charlton. When you reach the road, go left, and return to the pub.

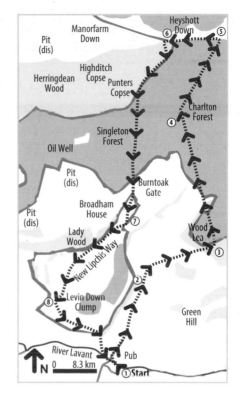

Points of interest

Levin Down is a Sussex Wildlife Trust Nature Reserve. The scrubby chalk grassland and heath allows for plenty of wildflowers and is an ideal habitat for butterflies.

Bosham and Fishbourne

START Bosham car park,
PO18 8HZ, SU806040

DISTANCE 6 miles (9.6km)

SUMMARY An easy flat walk along
mainly footpaths and a couple of
stretches of road. The beginning
section of the walk floods at high
tide so do check the tide times
before setting off (www.metoffice.
gov.uk/public/weather/tide-times)

PARKING Pay and display car park
at start point. Postcode: PO18 8HZ

MAPS OS Explorer OL8;
Landranger 197

WHERE TO EAT AND DRINK The
Bull's Head at the midway point
in Fishbourne (www.bulls-head-
fishbourne.co.uk) or the Anchor Bleu
at Bosham close to the start/end
point of the walk (anchorbleu.co.uk)

A circular walk between the coastal villages of Bosham and Fishbourne.

1   Leave the car park via the pedestrian access path left of the
toilets, then at the road turn right heading inland. When you reach the
Millstream Hotel turn left into the lane, follow it to the corner of the road
and take the public footpath straight ahead along an alleyway behind
houses. At the crossroads keep straight ahead until you reach the sea wall.

2   At the sea wall go left and walk along the shore for approximately ¼
mile (at low tide). When you reach a footpath up a couple of steps go left
and head towards the church. Follow the paved path as it leads you back
to the shoreline and continue walking, keeping the water to your right.
Follow the higher sea wall until you near a red post box by a bungalow,
then take the footpath here leading between houses to reach a road.

3   Cross over and climb the steps opposite and follow the footpath
across fields. The footpath leads on for just over ½ mile, passing a house
and then running alongside a barbed wire fence and finally reaches a road.

4   Cross over and continue straight ahead. You can see the spire of
Chichester cathedral ahead along this stretch. At the T-junction turn right
and walk up to the corner of the field, then turn left. You will soon arrive
at the Fishbourne Channel, home to many different species of seabirds.
Follow the path in a northerly direction along the water's edge. As you

near the tip of the Fishbourne Channel, the path takes you over a series of footbridges through reed beds before weaving behind houses and leading out to a lane.

5   At the lane go left. You will shortly arrive at the main road by the Bull's Head pub – turn left again. Follow the main road until you reach Old Park Lane. Go left here.

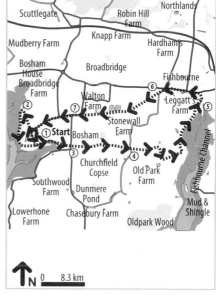

6   When you reach a junction with another road take the footpath leading into fields. Follow this straight ahead for 1 mile ignoring any turnings until you reach a road (Walton Lane).

7   At the road continue straight ahead following Walton Lane and then Bosham Lane back into the village. When you see the Millstream Hotel, bear left and walk back to the start point.

Points of interest

Bosham church is steeped in history. The Bayeux Tapestry portrays King Harold praying in Bosham church prior to his death in the Battle of Hastings in 1066.

Cissbury Ring

START Storrington Rise car park, BN14 0HT, TQ129076

DISTANCE 6 miles (9.5km) or 8½ miles (13.5km)

SUMMARY Two moderate walks following footpaths, bridleways and byways

PARKING Free car park at the start. Postcode: BN14 0HT

MAPS OS Explorer OL10; Landranger 198

WHERE TO EAT AND DRINK None en route

Two routes on the South Downs taking in far-reaching views and the largest hill fort in Sussex.

① Leave the car park and when the path immediately forks, go left. Follow the broad path uphill and bear left at the next fork. Follow the bridleway which swings right and then left through trees. Continue to a gate then follow the bridleway straight ahead through open countryside.

② When you near a lane go through two gates and take the chalky bridleway past a parking area leading away from Cissbury Ring. When the Monarch's Way crosses the bridleway, continue straight on ahead.

③ At the crossroads follow the restricted byway ahead. Remain on this path for 1 mile, bearing right at a fork nearly halfway along. Take a right-hand bridleway forking off the main path and follow it to the South Downs Way.

③a. For the shorter route turn right at the crossroads and follow the byway down to a junction. Rejoin the longer route at point 6.

④ At the South Downs Way go right and follow it for just over a mile to reach a crossroads. Ignore a left bridleway and a footpath into a field on the right as you walk this stretch.

⑤ At the crossroads turn right and follow the restricted byway (Monarch's Way). It soon heads downhill and reaches a junction after ¾ mile.

6 Take the grassy bridleway left (or right for the shorter route) and follow this bridleway through the valley for 1 mile to reach a T-junction with a gravel track.

7 Follow the byway right. Just past a barn take the left bridleway through a gate into Cissbury Ring. Bear left following the bridleway along the bottom edge of the wooded hillside with a wire fence to your left. At the gate turn sharp right. The path soon climbs steeply up to Cissbury Ring. Cross a chalk path and continue up then cross the next path and go through a gate to reach the hill fort.

8 Head towards the gap in the bank and then climb steps on the left. This leads you around the walls of the hill fort.

9 Take a set of stone steps leading down to a stile. Once over, head downhill and at the bottom go left. At a junction by a clearing take a path through a kissing gate on the right (signed for Findon Valley). You soon go through a gate on the right into access land. Bear left, winding down towards trees. Go through the gate and head directly across the path to another meadow. Go straight downhill then turn right through a gap in the hedge and head down to the car park.

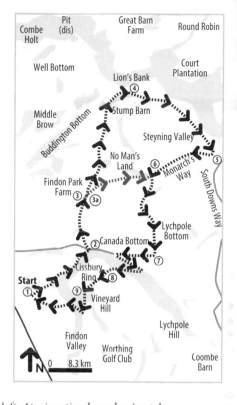

Points of interest

Cissbury Ring is an Iron Age hill fort and is the largest of its kind in Sussex.

Rudgwick

START Holy Trinity church,
Rudgwick, RH12 3EB, TQ090342

DISTANCE 6¼ miles (10km)

SUMMARY A moderate walk through
farmland along footpaths, bridleways
and lanes and a section of the Downs
Link; plenty of livestock along the way;
parts can be boggy after wet weather

PARKING Limited roadside
parking in Rudgwick by the
church. Postcode: RH12 3EB

MAPS OS Explorer OL34;
Landranger 187

WHERE TO EAT AND DRINK
The King's Head is at the start
and end point of the route
(kingsheadrudgwick.co.uk)

A walk on the border of West Sussex and Surrey taking in farmland, woodland
and a stretch of the Downs Link.

1   Starting with the church to your right walk straight ahead, then take
the Sussex Border Path down an alleyway on the left. Stick to the Sussex
Border Path, ignoring any footpath turnings, and continue through a gate.
The path soon leads into woods. At the fork go left and climb a stile into a
field.

2   The path skirts the field and leads to a stile. Cross the next field
keeping the former clay pit and fence to your left. Go through a gate
and turn right. Ignore the next right turning onto the Downs Link and
continue ahead on the footpath (Sussex Border Path) through the woods
to reach a stile into a field. Once across the field, take the footpath left.

3   Follow a broad farm track between fields. Ignore a right bridleway
turning by a house and continue ahead. Shortly, take a right footpath
leading through a gate into a small field, then through another gate
entering woodland.
     Once out of the woods the footpath skirts fields with trees to your left
before following a stream up to a main road.

4   Cross over and follow the footpath opposite through a kissing gate
and into fields. Turn left by a farmhouse following the footpath across the
field, then through two gates and down to a lane.

5 At the lane turn left. Walk approximately 150yds then take the right footpath over a stile. Walk along the right side of the field to a stile and then through a strip of woodland. The footpath leads to a brick bridge crossing the River Arun and then across another field. At a crossroads continue straight ahead to the road.

6 Cross over and walk a short distance along Naldretts Lane to a left footpath. This path leads through hedgerow, then across a field and past an old timber-framed house. At the T-junction turn right, then at the next junction go left and follow the clearly signed footpath through fields.

7 Just past a second footbridge into woods climb the stile on the right into a field. Follow the field's edge with woodland to your left to a gate opposite. Climb steps to the Downs Link.

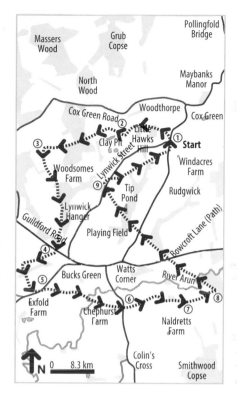

8 Turn left and follow the raised Downs Link path across the river and to a main road. Continue for another ¾ mile to a set of winding steps behind a bridge leading up to Lynwick Street.

9 Turn left into Lynwick Street and walk for around 100yds, then take the right-hand footpath into a field. Follow this signed footpath through fields and woodland to the start point. The path descends and then climbs a set of steps towards the end.

Points of interest

Rudgwick double bridge on the Downs Link. The two-tier railway bridge over the River Arun is made up of a brick arch on the bottom with an iron bridge built on top.

Stedham

START The village green, Stedham, GU29 0NQ, SU862223

DISTANCE 6¼ miles (10km)

SUMMARY An easy walk along footpaths, bridleways and lanes

PARKING Roadside parking at the start point. Postcode: GU29 0NQ

MAPS OS Explorer OL33; Landranger 197

WHERE TO EAT AND DRINK
The Hamilton Arms – Nava Thai is in the village of Stedham (thehamiltonarms.co.uk/the-pub)

A circular walk from Stedham taking in pine woodland, heathland and the River Rother.

1   Start with Stedham village green to your left then turn left into The Alley. Shortly take a right footpath through a gate into a field. Cross the field diagonally, bearing right to a tree-lined lane. Cross this and maintain direction across the next field. Descend steps to cross a road and a footbridge then head back up to reach a main road.

2   Cross over, turn right and walk for around 25yds to a lane on the left. Follow the lane uphill into woodland to reach a right-hand permissive footpath. Follow this through pinewoods for approximately ¼ mile until it bends left and reaches a crossroads. Go right and head downhill to reach a T-junction. Turn left. At the next crossroads go right and then walk ahead to another crossroads (staggered) and go right again. Continue along the footpath, bearing right when it forks, to reach a lane.

3   Turn right and then almost immediately right again following the footpath along a drive to a fork. Bear right and head back into woodland to reach a T-junction. Go right and walk downhill to cross a footbridge and then cross a field. Climb a stile and continue along the right-hand side of fields to a farm. Go through a gate and walk past a house, then follow the path to Minsted Road.

4   Turn right and walk to a left bridleway following a lane. After around 300yds, at the T-junction, go left. Walk for just under ¼ mile heading back into woodland to reach another T-junction, go left. Follow the tree-lined

bridleway forking right by a house. Remain on this path ignoring a right bridleway and continuing over a driveway and through woods to where the path forks again. Go right and walk downhill for approximately 200yds to a road.

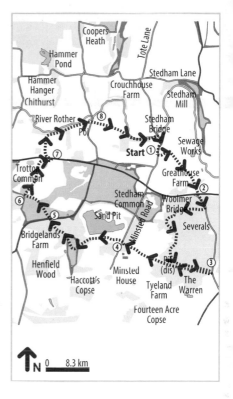

⑤ Cross Elsted Road and take the bridleway opposite into Iping Common. You soon reach a crossroads; keep straight ahead here, and again when another track crosses the bridleway. Head uphill and once at the top, fork right. Shortly at a crossroads turn right.

⑥ Follow this bridleway, continuing straight ahead when another path crosses it. After around ⅓ mile, follow the path to the right and then left and to a busy road.

⑦ Turn left at the road then take the next right. Walk past a garage and follow the footpath across a meadow to reach a T-junction. Turn right over a stile. Cross the next meadow to another stile and enter a small area of woodland. The footpath leads over a stream and skirts another field before arriving at Iping Lane.

⑧ Cross and take the bridleway opposite. Pass a cottage and bear right then follow the bridleway for just over ½ mile as it leads across farmland and into woods and runs alongside the River Rother. When you arrive back at Stedham, turn right and follow The Street back to the start point.

Points of interest

The tiny village of Iping is the setting for much of H. G. Wells' science fiction story, *The Invisible Man*.

Boxgrove and Halnaker

START Boxgrove village hall car park, PO18 0EE, SU906075

DISTANCE 6¼ miles (10km)

SUMMARY A moderate walk on footpaths, bridleways, lanes and one short stretch of busy road

PARKING Free car park at the start point. Postcode: PO18 0EE

MAPS OS Explorer OL10; Landranger 197

WHERE TO EAT AND DRINK The Anglesey Arms is close to the start and end point (theangleseyarms.com)

A varied walk taking in a windmill and the ruins of a monastery along the way.

① From Boxgrove village hall turn left and head uphill, then cross over the road and take the right footpath. At a T-junction turn left and follow the footpath round the field, then fork right. Follow the tree-lined footpath through Tinwood Vineyard to reach a lane. Turn right and after around 100yds take the footpath left.

② Follow the clearly signed footpath through fields, eventually arriving at a gate leading out to the main road. Cross to the parking bays and information board.

③ Go right, taking the track signed for Halnaker Windmill through the tunnel of trees. The path continues on the right-hand side along a raised bank to reach a fork in the path. Go left here to visit the windmill.

④ Retrace your steps back down and turn left. Follow the path for just under ¼ mile passing another vineyard to reach a stile by a track. Climb the stile and follow the path ahead keeping a fence to your right. This leads to a gap in the hedge and shortly to another field. Cross the field, following the path in line with pylons to a road.

⑤ Turn left and walk along the grass verge, then just after gates to Selhurst Park cross and take the right footpath into woodland. After around 200yds cross a stile and farm track and continue straight ahead. This leads to a large field. Head uphill then once at the top, head down to the bottom right corner of the field.

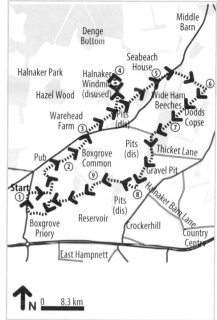

6 Go right. The footpath leads diagonally back uphill across the next field heading towards a copse of trees. At the top turn left and walk along the bottom edge of the copse, then walk diagonally across the next field to the right-hand corner.

7 Turn right into woodland and shortly reach a three-way fingerpost. Go left and follow the path down to Thicket Lane. Turn left, then when the road swings left, take the bridleway right, back into woodland. Continue to reach a farm track, cross this and continue on the bridleway opposite to reach Tinwood Lane.

8 Turn right. Walk past paddocks to where the tarmac runs out by a gate and Tinwood Lane forks right. Follow this track heading through the trees. Ignore the first left kissing gate, then take the left footpath through the next kissing gate.

9 Go right and follow the path past a line of trees. Keep straight ahead at a crossroads continuing to a T-junction. Turn left and follow the path running alongside a hedgerow then when the hedgerow runs out, go right. This leads through a kissing gate and onto Church Lane. Turn right and return to Boxgrove village hall.

Points of interest

Boxgrove Priory was built in the twelfth century and destroyed in the sixteenth century during the Dissolution of the Monasteries.
Halnaker Windmill is thought to date back to the late eighteenth century. The recently restored windmill was struck by lightning in 1905.

Arundel

START Mill Road, Arundel,
BN18 9PA, TQ020071

DISTANCE 6⅓ miles (10.2km)
or 8¼ miles (13.3km)

SUMMARY Two moderate walks on
footpaths, bridleways and roadside;
much of it is riverside walking –
can be muddy, some cattle

PARKING Large pay and display
car park or roadside parking at the
start point. Postcode: BN18 9PA

MAPS OS Explorer OL10;
Landranger 197

WHERE TO EAT AND DRINK The
Black Rabbit pub is passed on both
routes (theblackrabbitarundel.co.uk)

Two walks around the stunning downland countryside by Arundel Castle and
Swanbourne Lake.

(1) Facing Arundel Castle, turn right and walk along Mill Road. After
around 175yds take a path on the right past some tennis courts. Follow
the bridleway ahead, ignoring a right turning until you reach the river.

(2) Climb the bank and turn left. When you reach a sluice where a
stream meets the Arun keep straight ahead, ignoring two footpaths
leading left. Continue along the riverbank as it passes behind the Wildfowl
and Wetlands reserve and leads to the Black Rabbit pub. Take the road
heading uphill behind the pub and at the top turn left. Walk for 50yds,
then take a right bridleway.

(3) Follow the bridleway downhill and then across a field. Continue
straight on along this path for almost ½ mile. It swings left and then
arrives at a lane by the hamlet of South Stoke.

(4) Take the bridleway opposite along a farm drive and then round to the
left. Once past the farm continue straight ahead. The bridleway descends
to a gate and then follows the edge of a field and leads uphill. Once out of
the field, follow the path down as it winds through trees to the riverbank.
Continue along this bridleway for around ⅓ mile.

(5) Enter Arundel Park and follow the footpath left as it heads uphill.
The path bends round to the right and soon after forks. Take the left-hand
fork and continue to climb steeply up. Once at the top, climb the stile and

then follow the footpath over the hill. When the path forks, go right and follow the path as it leads downhill to another stile. Cross the field and continue down remaining on this path for around ½ mile.

⑥ When you reach a junction, bear left and follow the footpath through the valley to a gate into Swanbourne Lake. Take the path leading left and follow it around the edge of the lake until you reach the gated entrance by a cafe.

⑦a. For the shorter route leave the park and turn right onto Mill Road heading over the bridge and back to the start.

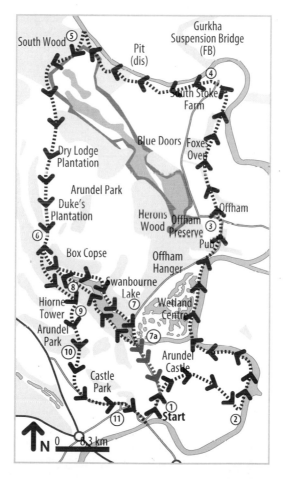

7 For the longer route go through the gate and follow Mill Road a short distance then bear right to follow the path all the way along the other side of Swanbourne Lake.

8 Once you've looped the lake follow the footpath over the stile and back through the valley. When you get back to the junction you met at point 6, turn sharp left and head uphill enjoying the views as you climb. Continue ahead to reach a gate.

9 Just after the gate and stile turn right, heading up through trees. This leads up to open parkland and past the Hiorne Tower. Bear left across the grass to reach a tarmac path.

10 Turn left and follow the path down to park gates. Walk straight ahead to London Road, then turn left and walk past Arundel Cathedral to reach Arundel Castle gates.

11 Follow the road round to the right and head down the high street. Continue straight ahead on the left-hand side until you reach Mill Road. Turn left and head back to the start.

Kithurst Hill

START Kithurst Hill car park,
RH20 4HW, TQ070125

DISTANCE 6¾ miles (10.8km)

SUMMARY A moderate route mainly
along bridleways; some hills

PARKING Free car park at the start
point. Postcode: RH20 4HW

MAPS OS Explorer OL10;
Landranger 197

WHERE TO EAT AND
DRINK None en route

This circular route high up on the South Downs provides far-reaching views
across West Sussex.

1   From the car park entrance walk across the grass opposite and take
the bridleway leading gradually uphill. When you come to a crossroads
with another bridleway continue straight ahead. Just past a trig point a
bridleway goes off to the right, ignore this and continue on the same path
through a gate and then down through a field ignoring another bridleway
turning on the left. Continue walking to reach another gate and Chantry
Lane.

2   Turn right onto Chantry Lane and climb the hill to reach a junction
with the South Downs Way and a parking area. From here, pass the metal
gate, then follow the bridleway ahead leading downhill. Continue along
this bridleway for just over a mile to reach Michelgrove Lane.

3   When you arrive at a set of metal gates by a barn, go right and follow
Michelgrove Lane to a farm. Once past the farm and houses, ignore a
bridleway turning on the right and head uphill. After approximately
¾ mile a bridleway goes off to the left. Ignore this and walk for around
another 100yds to reach a T-junction where the bridleway splits.

4   Go right here and follow the wide chalky bridleway, ignoring a
turning off to the left after a short distance. Remain on the bridleway for
just over 1 mile, ignoring any turnings going off either side, as it heads
through a gate and uphill through hedgerow until you eventually arrive at
a staggered crossroads.

[5] When you reach the crossroads turn right, walk a few paces, then turn left onto the bridleway. Remain on this bridleway (ignoring a turning on the left) following it through a bushy area and then along the left-hand side of a field. After approximately ⅓ mile you will arrive back at the South Downs Way.

[6] Turn right onto the South Downs Way and follow it uphill. Continue following the South Downs Way for 1¼ miles (ignoring a right-hand bridleway turning not long after the trig point at the top of Rackham Hill) taking in the stunning panoramic views, until you arrive back at Kithurst Hill car park.

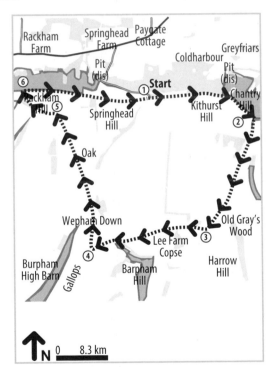

Points of interest

Kithurst Hill is almost at the halfway point of the 100-mile-long South Downs Way. The route offers spectacular views over the South Downs, nearby Amberley Wild Brooks and out to sea.

Loxwood

START The Canal Centre,
Loxwood, RH14 0RD, TQ041311

DISTANCE 6¾ miles (10.8km)

SUMMARY An easy walk along
the canal towpath, footpaths,
bridleways and lanes

PARKING Car park by the
start. Postcode: RH14 0RD

MAPS OS Explorer OL34;
Landranger 186

WHERE TO EAT AND DRINK The
Onslow Arms pub is by the start
(onslowarmsloxwood.com)

A walk along the border of West Sussex and Surrey taking in the restored Wey
and Arun Canal at Loxwood.

1   Starting at the information centre, walk past the pub and under a
bridge. Follow the bridleway alongside the restored section of the Wey
and Arun Canal for just over 1 mile, ignoring any footpath turnings off
the towpath. Just past Southlands Lock continue ahead on the bridleway
as it follows the course of an unrestored section of the canal. After around
⅓ mile you will reach Gennets Bridge Lock. Turn right onto the Sussex
Border Path crossing the canal.

2   Follow the path to a crossroads where you keep straight ahead. Once
past a farm, head downhill to a gate and then continue along the signed
Sussex Border Path as it follows Oakhurst Lane to reach a main road.

3   At Guildford Road turn left, walk for approximately 100yds, then
turn right onto Pigbush Lane. Follow the Sussex Border Path along the
lane for around ½ mile as it leads uphill to a crossroads. Go straight ahead
here walking down to a farm and then through a gate. The bridleway takes
you through woodland to a footpath on the right.

4   Turn right onto this footpath and walk through the woods, ignoring
a turning on the right after around 200yds. When the footpath meets a
bridleway, go right and follow the bridleway as it bends round, ignoring a
footpath turning on the right and another on the left as you walk. Climb a
small hill then when the bridleway forks take the clearly defined path right
and follow it for almost ½ mile to a road.

⑤ At Loxwood Road turn right, walk a few paces, then cross over and take the footpath opposite. The path leads past a farm and into woodland, then meets a wide track leading to a crossroads. At the crossroads go right to reach another crossroads. Go left here and pass a pond, then go left again and follow the footpath to a lane.

⑥ At Drungewick Lane turn right. Follow the lane as it winds down to cross a stream and shortly after cross the Drungewick Lane Canal bridge. Turn right onto the canal towpath, then follow it for just over 1½ miles as it meanders back to the Canal Centre.

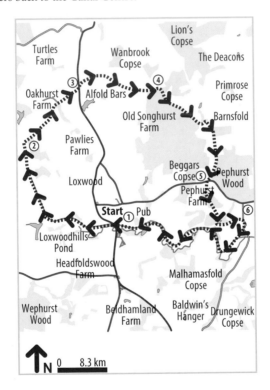

Points of interest

The Wey and Arun Canal: work has been ongoing since the 1970s to restore the nineteenth-century canal, which was first opened in 1816 and then closed in 1871 after the introduction of railways led to its demise.

Sidlesham Quay

START Pagham Harbour RSPB Visitor
Centre, PO20 7NE, SZ856967

DISTANCE 6¾ miles (10.7km)

SUMMARY A moderate walk along
shoreline and farmland footpaths
and lanes; parts of this route are
only accessible at low tide, for
tide times: www.metoffice.gov.
uk/public/weather/tide-times/

PARKING Free car park at the visitor
centre. Postcode: PO20 7NE

MAPS OS Explorer OL08;
Landranger 197

WHERE TO EAT AND DRINK The
Crab and Lobster at Sidlesham
Quay (crab-lobster.co.uk)

A walk exploring the western shoreline of Pagham Harbour around Sidlesham
Quay and Church Norton.

1 From the car park follow the path past the RSPB visitor centre in
the direction of the harbour. Shortly take a footpath on the left signed for
Yeoman's Field.

The path swings round by a pool and then goes left again leading
through hedgerow to a field. Follow the path along the left edge of the field
until it narrows and leads to houses. Continue to the gate (ignoring a right
footpath turning) and walk past houses to a lane.

2 Turn right and follow the quiet road ahead to Sidlesham Quay.
Continue along Mill Lane as it bends left, passing the Crab and Lobster
pub. After approximately 200yds take a footpath on the right and follow it
to the edge of Pagham Harbour.

3 At the harbour turn right (this section can only be walked at low
tide). Follow the path as it winds its way along the shoreline leading back
to Sidlesham Quay and the corner of Mill Lane. Continue back along the
lane then take the path on the left signed for the visitor centre.

4 Follow the path along the harbour's edge, ignoring any turnings
off. After just over ½ mile you will get to a turning for the visitor centre.
Ignore this and keep straight ahead for around another ½ mile along the
shore. The path swings right at the Ferry Channel and then crosses it with
a turn to the left.

5 Continue along the shoreline path towards Church Norton. After nearly 1½ miles, there is a footpath turning on the right. Ignore this and continue straight ahead to explore the headland (at low tide).

6 Take the next footpath on the right. This leads down through trees and then through a field to a T-junction. Turn right and follow the footpath past a farmhouse. Continue straight ahead following the track through an industrial area leading to Rectory Lane.

7 Turn right and follow Rectory Lane to the end, then go left, walking up to St Wilfred's church. Once in the car park, take the footpath past a gate leading back to the shoreline. Turn left and walk back along the shoreline path.

8 After crossing Ferry Channel go straight ahead taking the path into the RSPB centre. Follow the main path through the reserve, back to the start point.

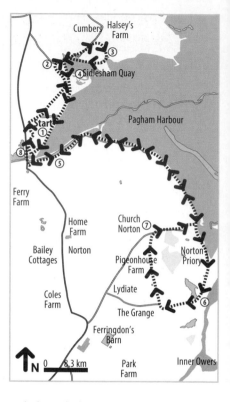

Points of interest

St Wilfred's at Church Norton is well worth a visit. The remaining church building was the chancel of a much larger Norman church, which was dismantled and rebuilt in nearby Selsey during the 1860s.

Balcombe

START The Half Moon Inn, Haywards Heath Road, RH17 6PA, TQ309306

DISTANCE 7 miles (11km)

SUMMARY A moderate walk following footpaths, bridleways and lanes

PARKING Roadside parking near the start. Postcode: RH17 6PA

MAPS OS Explorer 135; Landranger 187

WHERE TO EAT AND DRINK The Half Moon Inn, Balcombe is at the start and end point (halfmoonbalcombe.com)

An interesting route from the village of Balcombe taking in a stretch of Ardingly Reservoir and passing Wakehurst Place.

1   Walk to the end of the small road to the right of the pub. Take the footpath left across a field. This leads to woods with a boardwalk section over a stream and to a T-junction where you go right (ignore a right footpath turning just before the stream). Follow the footpath along a track for nearly ½ mile, to reach a stone bridge with a staggered junction either side.

2   Keep straight ahead following the track through woodland. Stick to the main footpath for just over ½ mile ignoring any forestry track turnings as you go. Continue to the road.

3   At the lane turn left and walk for around 100yds to a right footpath turning. Climb a stile and head down past Little Strudgate Farm, then follow the track as it weaves through woodland, passes a pond and follows another stream. Follow the track as it climbs and emerges from the woods to reach Newhouse Farm.

4   At the farm cottages, take the footpath right. Go through the gate and head towards the woods. At the top of the field follow the footpath with trees to your right, then at the corner of the next field climb the stile and walk through the woodland. Follow the path downhill and cross a stream, then when you reach a T-junction, go right. Continue along this footpath for around ½ mile to Wakehurst Place.

5 At the T-junction with a lane in Wakehurst Place turn right. Follow the lane, then take a footpath to the left of the Millennium Seed Bank. The lane then becomes a track, which you leave at a right turn to go straight ahead and across a field down to woodland. Follow it round to the right and cross a farm track. Cross Ardingly Brook via footbridges and then continue steeply up through woodland. When you emerge the path skirts the woods and leads to a stile onto Paddockhurst Lane.

6 Turn left and follow the lane for just over ½ mile. When the road forks go right, following Mill Lane towards Edmond's Farm. Walk for around 200yds then turn left, taking the bridleway bearing right off the farm track almost immediately and leading down to Ardingly Reservoir.

7 At the reservoir, turn right and follow the bridleway along the water's edge. This leads to woodland and then to Mill Lane. Turn left and follow the road across the reservoir.

8 Once across the water follow the road to the top of a hill where the road bends sharply left and shortly take a footpath on the right over a stile. Follow the path across a stream and past woodland to a T-junction. Turn left and walk gently uphill across fields and along a track back to the start point.

Points of interest

The Millennium Seed Bank. Part of Wakehurst Place, the giant seed bank houses a collection of more than 2.4 billion seeds from across the globe.

Thorney Island

START Thornham Lane,
PO10 8DD, SU756049

DISTANCE 7 miles (11km)

SUMMARY A moderate walk following
the Sussex Border Path around the
island, this coastal route is best done
at low tide so do check the tide times
before setting off: www.metoffice.
gov.uk/public/weather/tide-times/

PARKING Small free car park at the
start point where Thorney Road meets
Thornham Lane. Postcode: PO10 8DD

MAPS OS Explorer OL08;
Landranger 197

WHERE TO EAT AND
DRINK None en route

Get away from it all on this remote circular walk around a military base on the border with Hampshire.

① From the car park entrance, turn left onto Thornham Lane. At the marina go straight ahead past houses and between two large rocks and continue towards the shoreline.

② At Thornham Point turn left and then shortly after go right following the footpath over a wooden bridge. Remain on the Sussex Border Path, which you follow all the way around the peninsula.

③ When you arrive at some slightly intimidating looking security gates you need to buzz and wait to be let through. To access Thorney Island and all it has to offer, you will need to be given access by the Ministry of Defence who own the land. Walkers are usually let straight through but occasionally can be asked for details such as name and address. Once through the gates you must stick to the clearly marked path as you walk.

④ After approximately 1 mile the path heads up the bank towards the thirteenth-century church of St Nicholas. The church is open for visitors and can be accessed via some steps leading into the churchyard. At the Thorney Island Sailing Club (TISC) there are two options as the shoreline footpath can flood at high tide. At low tide take the shoreline path but if the water is high take the alternative route behind the sailing club, which then leads back to rejoin the shoreline path.

[5] When you reach the southern tip of Thorney Island there is a glorious sandy beach. This is Pilsey Island, an RSPB reserve. Remain on the footpath for just over a mile where there are benches if you want to stop for a picnic.

[6] The path leads you to Marker Point where seals can sometimes be spotted and then continues to wind along the west of the peninsula with more glorious views. When you reach a second security gate by the Great Deep, press the buzzer and as before wait to be let through, then continue along the waterside path.

[7] As you near some chalets and Emsworth Marina, take the first footpath on the right. Follow this past paddocks and through a farm and back to the start point of the walk.

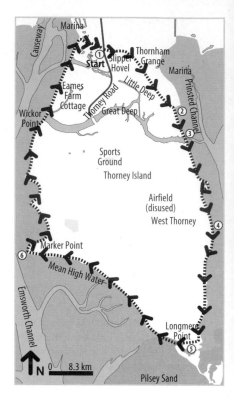

Points of interest

At St Nicholas church there are a number of war graves including those of German soldiers killed during the Second World War. In total there are fifty-two Commonwealth war graves in the churchyard as well as the graves of twenty-one German Air Force men.

Arun Valley 2

START Amberley Rail Station, BN18 9LR, TQ026118

DISTANCE 7 miles (11.3km)

SUMMARY A linear walk on bridleways and footpaths between two rail stations; can get very muddy and wet

PARKING Car park at Amberley station. Postcode: BN18 9LR

MAPS OS Explorer OL10; Landranger 197

WHERE TO EAT AND DRINK The Bridge Inn is close to the start point (www.bridgeinnamberley.com)

A linear walk between Amberley and Pulborough rail stations, alongside the River Arun and through the Arun valley.

1   Leave Amberley station, cross the road and walk under the railway bridge. Once under the bridge turn right onto a footpath leading to the banks of the river. Keep to the riverbank path, ignoring turnings off for approximately 1 mile. When you arrive level with the village of Bury on the opposite side of the river, turn right.

2   Cross the meadow to a gate then follow the path over a ditch and a stile. Continue through a series of fields to reach a railway track. Cross this and follow the footpath past the ruins of Amberley Castle to reach Amberley village. Walk straight ahead along Church Street to reach Hog Lane on the left. Take this and walk for approximately 100yds, then take a left-hand footpath downhill through a gate.

3   Follow the footpath into Amberley Wild Brooks and continue for approximately 1 mile through the nature reserve. When you arrive at a gate by an information board continue straight ahead towards woodland. Once through the scrubby woodland cross two footbridges and continue ahead towards a house. The footpath leads through two gates and soon through a farm. Once through the farmyard remain on the track for around 350yds, then go left following the footpath past hedges and along the riverbank towards Greatham Bridge.

4 Turn left at the lane, crossing the bridge, then continue along the lane to reach a right-hand footpath. Take this and follow the path to reach a main road.

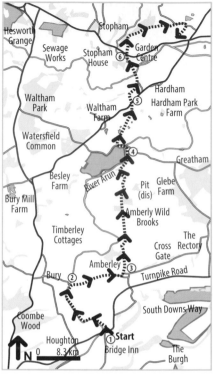

5 Turn right and take the footpath a little further along on the opposite side of the road, which leads across a field and over the railway line. Cross the next field, go through a gate and follow the path right. At the access road to a pumping station go left at the T-junction. Walk past the Southern Water site then cross the river. The footpath leads you through a field to another river bridge. Cross this then walk to the road.

6 Cross over and follow the footpath opposite to reach a T-junction with a bridleway. Go right and continue along this for around ⅓ mile.

Just past a cottage and farmhouse, the bridleway joins a drive. Continue straight ahead here taking a footpath leading through bushes and across fields towards Pulborough church. When you arrive at a road, go right and follow the lane as it crosses the railway before turning right onto a footpath leading to Pulborough station.

Points of interest

Amberley Castle dates back to the twelfth century and was used by the Bishops of Chichester for nearly 400 years. It was a loyalist stronghold during the English Civil War until Cromwell ordered its destruction in 1643. In 1660 King Charles II returned it to the Bishopric. Since the 1980s it has been a luxury hotel.

Rake

START National Trust car park for Durford Wood, GU31 5DS, SU790259

DISTANCE 7¼ miles (11.7km)

SUMMARY A moderate walk following footpaths, bridleways, lanes and road

PARKING National Trust car park at the start. Postcode: GU31 5DS

MAPS OS Explorer OL33; Landranger 197

WHERE TO EAT AND DRINK The Flying Bull Inn in Rake (theflyingbull.com)

Take a walk right on the border of West Sussex and Hampshire through tranquil woodland enjoying downland views.

1   From the car park take the bridleway through the gate. The path initially goes straight ahead and then turns left. Follow the wide bridleway (Sussex Border Path) through the trees, remaining straight ahead when another path crosses it.

When the path forks go right, remaining on the Sussex Border Path as it leads uphill and then down past a field.

2   At the bottom of the hill take the footpath left. Follow the path up past a house, then at the T-junction turn left. Head through the trees, ignoring a right footpath into a field. The bridleway swings right as the trees open out and runs between fences. At the end turn left and then almost immediately right.

3   Follow the bridleway ignoring a left permissive footpath turning. At the T-junction go left and continue through the pine woodland. When the path forks go left, remaining on the bridleway. At the four-way junction turn sharp right onto the footpath leading downhill.

4   Follow the waymarked public footpath straight ahead through Rogate Common, ignoring any permissive footpaths going off to the left or right. When the path forks go left and continue until you reach the road.

5   Go left and follow the road (taking care as there is little verge) to reach a right-hand lane signed for Chithurst. Take this and walk for around 175yds, then turn left onto a bridleway leading between fences.

⑥ Follow the bridleway down into woodland. Cross a track and continue straight ahead as the bridleway runs between fences through the Fyning Hill Estate and eventually reaches a road.

⑦ Turn right and follow the road for ¼ mile. Just before you reach large gates to a house, take a left footpath over a footbridge and stile (easy to miss). Follow the path along the edge of the field then climb the stile and take the right footpath into trees, ignoring the left footpath over a footbridge. The path leads to Combe Pond and out to a quiet lane.

⑧ Follow quiet Canhouse Lane left for nearly a mile.

⑨ When you get to the end of the lane, turn right, then almost immediately left onto a footpath (Sussex Border Path) leading past houses. Remain on the Sussex Border Path as it takes you through Rake Hanger, ignoring any footpaths on the left or right. The path joins a road leading down to another. Turn left onto Rogate Road, walk past cottages, then turn right into the car park.

Points of interest

 Rake Hanger is a Site of Special Scientific Interest (SSSI). The ancient woodland was designated nationally important due to the sessile oaks and alder woodland found there.

Lavant and the Trundle

START The Earl of March pub, Lavant, PO18 oBQ, SU857082

DISTANCE 7½ miles (12km)

SUMMARY A moderate walk along footpaths, bridleways and byways and lanes

PARKING Roadside parking by the start point. Postcode: PO18 oBQ

MAPS OS Explorer OLo8; Landranger 197

WHERE TO EAT AND DRINK The Earl of March pub is at the start and end point (theearlofmarch.com)

This route follows a disused railway line before climbing to an Iron Age hill fort with spectacular views.

① With your back to the Earl of March pub, turn right and begin walking along the main road. Just before you get to Sheepwash Lane take a footpath on the left along an alleyway signed for the Centurion Way. Head right at the Centurion Way in the direction of West Dean and follow the surfaced path under two old railway bridges to reach a residential area. Keep straight ahead and pass a play park on the right, then once at the end of the road (Churchmead Close), cross over and maintain direction until you reach a green. Bear right following the path diagonally across the green, then rejoin the next clear section of the Centurion Way.

② Remain on the surfaced path of the Centurion Way for almost 2 miles as it passes through peaceful countryside leading up to West Dean.

③ When you reach a set of steps on the right, climb these and turn right at the road. Walk past West Dean Primary School to the main road, then cross over and continue ahead along the lane opposite. At the end of the road turn right, walk for a short distance to cross a small bridge over the River Lavant and then turn right again. Follow this bridleway (part of the Monarch's Way) alongside a wall belonging to West Dean House and Gardens. Continue along the Monarch's Way and when the path forks with another bridleway, go left heading uphill into woodland.

④ When you arrive at a road by a house and a car park, cross over and follow the bridleway opposite leading up to the Trundle, the remains of an Iron Age hill fort. The path takes you up and loops you around the Trundle and is well worth the climb for the amazing views. Bear right, ignoring any turnings off and once around head back in the same direction you came from towards the car park. Once back at the road turn left and begin following the wide byway (Chalkpit Lane) downhill.

⑤ Follow the chalky byway for 1½ miles straight ahead down to Lavant, taking in the views as you go.

⑥ When you reach Pook Lane turn right and walk through the village bearing right into Sheepwash Lane when the road forks. Follow this up to the main road, then turn left and head back to the pub.

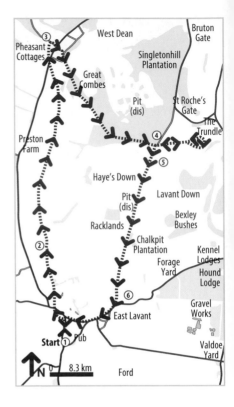

Points of interest

The Trundle is an ancient Iron Age hill fort which was created at least 6,000 years ago. Its name comes from the Old English word Tryndle, meaning circle.

Bepton

START Bepton Road,
GU29 0JB, SU860181

DISTANCE 8 miles (12.9km)

SUMMARY A moderate walk
along footpaths, bridleways,
byways and lanes

PARKING Limited roadside
parking on Bepton Road by the
start point. Postcode: GU29 0JB

MAPS OS Explorer OL08;
Landranger 197

WHERE TO EAT AND
DRINK None en route

A gorgeous varied walk through countryside and woodland with spectacular
views from the South Downs Way.

[1] Starting by the junction of two lanes with the Bepton Down
noticeboard to your left, cross over and follow the restricted byway
opposite. Take the first bridleway turning on the right and follow the path
as it winds uphill around the wooded hillside, getting steeper as you climb.
At the top go through a gate and bear right across the field. Go through
another gate and turn right.

[2] Follow the South Downs Way for just over 1½ miles, ignoring a
byway and a bridleway on the right as you walk. Ignore a right-hand
footpath and just past this the Devil's Jumps appear. A footpath leads
you to see the Bronze Age burial mounds just after passing them. After
viewing them, return to the South Downs Way and continue on.

[3] When you reach a crossroads, go left following a footpath into a field.
The footpath runs along the right side of the field, then heads down a
short hill and swings right. Follow the path through the valley.

[4] When you reach a farm building ignore a right-hand grassy footpath
and continue along the same clearly defined path as it swings round
and leads uphill. You soon head into the trees. Continue along this path
ignoring any turnings for just over ¾ mile until you reach a lane.

[5] At the lane turn left. Where the road bends ignore a left turning and
instead continue along the quiet lane as it swings right. Walk to where the
lane forks, then go left following the sign for West Dean and head uphill.

6 Take the left bridleway and follow it along the left side of a meadow and into West Dean Woods. There are large boulders (an art installation) dotted along the bridleway as you walk straight ahead through the woodland. Ignore a right bridleway after around a mile, then just after this go right at the fork continuing with tall trees to your left.

7 At the crossroads by another large boulder remain straight ahead for approximately ⅓ mile. At the South Downs Way turn right and continue to a crossroads.

8 Take the left byway downhill. Ignore a gate halfway down and continue walking to reach a bridleway on the left. Take this and follow it downhill back to Bepton.

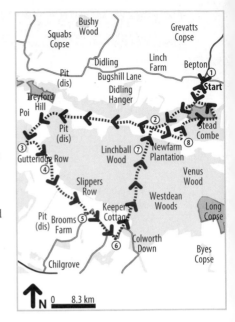

Points of interest

The Devil's Jumps are five Bronze Age burial mounds, constructed around 3,500 years ago. They are located just off the South Downs Way and are clearly visible.

West Itchenor and West Wittering

START The Street, West Itchenor, PO20 7AH, SU799013

DISTANCE 8½ miles (13.7km)

SUMMARY A moderate walk along footpaths, beach and roads; some of this route should be done at low tide so do check the tide times (www.metoffice.gov.uk/public/weather/tide-times/)

PARKING Itchenor pay and display car park close to the start point. Postcode: PO20 7AE

MAPS OS Explorer OL08; Landranger 197

WHERE TO EAT AND DRINK The Landing Coffee Shop is on Pound Road (www.facebook.com/thelandingcoffeeshop)

A seaside route between West Itchenor and West Wittering and around the sand dune spit of East Head.

1 Follow The Street south for approximately ⅓ mile until you come to the corner of the road. Leave the road here and take the path signed for Salterns Way, which leads behind Itchenor Memorial Hall and heads through fields. The footpath crosses a lane and then continues through fields to reach a T-junction.

2 At the T-junction, turn right and follow the Salterns Way for ½ mile, ignoring a footpath on the left as you go. Continue on until you reach a main road.

3 Go right at Rockwood Lane and follow it for just over ½ mile until you reach the shops of West Wittering. Walk through the seaside village and turn right into Pound Road.

4 Walk a short distance and then, immediately past a toilet block, take a lane on the left signed for West Wittering beach. Continue all the way down to the beach car park.

5 Walk onto the beach then turn right and walk alongside the beach huts. Continue along the beach, walking all the way around East Head. The sand dune spit offers great coastal views and is home to birds such as little egrets, lapwings and curlews.

6 Once around East Head walk back towards the car park on the Chichester Harbour side. Follow the footpath to the left of the car park, which leads you to the sea wall. Follow the shoreline path enjoying the views over Chichester Harbour and ignoring any right turns as you go.

7 The path briefly heads inland to wind around some houses at one point along this almost 3-mile long stretch but otherwise continues along the water's edge, offering gorgeous views over the harbour. Just after a boardwalk, a footpath goes off to the right – ignore this and remain on the shoreline path. When you get to a boatyard keep straight ahead and follow the public footpath back to West Itchenor and The Street where the walk began.

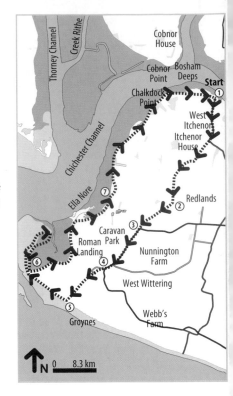

Points of interest

East Head is a sand dune and shingle spit, managed by the National Trust. The area provides a rich habitat for a wide variety of birds and wildlife and is designated a Site of Special Scientific Interest (SSSI). As well as an ever-changing population of birds, the area is home to seals, lizards and many wildflowers.